Other books by John D. Forlini:

Acid Reflux; Options for Controlling & Conquering
Algebra; A Mini Book Overview for High Schooler's and Others
Geometry; A Mini Book Overview for High Schooler's and Others
Chemistry; A Mini Book Overview for High Schooler's and Others
Physics; A Mini Book Overview for High Schooler's and Others
Trigonometry; A Mini Book Overview for High Schooler's and Others
Calculus; A Mini Book Overview for High Schooler's and Others
Eighth Grade Common Core Math
How to Get A's in High School Math and Science
The 1930's; Road from the Past, Portal to the Future
Murder; Old Time Murder Mystery
Workbook for Eighth Grade Common Core Math
Longevity; Living to120 and Beyond and Enjoying the Ride

Other writings by John D. Forlini:

Journal of Chromatographic Science *Separation of Glycol, Methanol, and Small Quantities of Diethylene Glycol by Gas Liquid Chromatography.*

Today's Industrial Products & Solutions *PLC Versus DCS: Does a Distinction Really Exist Anymore?*

Dedication

This book is dedicated to the brave souls in this book who let me interview and write their retirement stories and life biography.

Publisher: 4lini Publishing; Alabama.
4linipublishing@charter.net

ISBN 13: 978-1974577835
ISBN 10: 197457783X

Disclaimer: This is not a medical manual. The information provided is to help retirees be aware of the available literature and options with which to make intelligent decisions. It is not intended as a substitute for any treatment that might have been prescribed by ones doctor or the normal process of deciding when to see a doctor. If you believe you have a medical issue or problem, I urge you to seek medical help. Any use of this book is at the reader's discretion. Mention of specific products or brand names does not imply endorsement either by me or by the makers as an endorsement of me. Discussion of remedies, tests, surgical procedures, foods, and or medical procedures and doctors does not mean endorsement or suggest that any of these are recommended or not recommended.

Note to fellow septuagenarians, and to those younger and older,

While this book has been edited and edited, there is always something that could be missed or added to improve.

The beauty of Amazon.com is that they only publish on demand. That is they only publish when a book is ordered. Thus an author can make a change digitally and the next book will have this change.

So, if you should find something you feel needs correcting, or included please email to:

4linipublishing@charter.net

The needed change will be made within 24-48 hours and you will be acknowledged on this page for your contribution as follows:

Contributor   Date Contributed   Date Corrected

No corrections or additions are included to date.

RETIREMENT

Nine Recent Biographies

Plus Appropriate Recent Literature

Prescription for Happy Retirement

By John D. Forlini

Table of Contents

Purpose of this Book

The overall purpose of this book is to provide the information and tools to enable each individual to improve his or her retirement life and life span. By reading about what others have done, greater insight can be obtained. From taking in renters, to obtaining reverse mortgages, to investing wisely, to proper handling of real estate these retirees have used every available means at their disposal to remain alive and active. This book provides their biography's and insight and activities. The final chapter incorporates these biographies with recent literature to provide a blueprint for retirement.

No two people have exactly the same financial, age, marital status, travel plans, desires, health, enjoyable activities, and goals for retirement. But, by examining the nine people in this book who have either retired, are in process of retiring, or have been retired for several decades you can learn many valuable lessons. This book also incorporates recent writings and research on retirement to enhance the nine real life case histories. If for instance someone is contemplating a reverse mortgage, then this is a must read.

The author of this book is 74 years of age and has retired and/or been retired by the companies he worked for four times. Currently, I am working (part time) for a company that does high tech industrial controls integration. I plan to retire in the coming year--again. It might sound like the author is well off- but in fact he and his wife just get by.

The nine people in this book were selected because of their eclectic backgrounds. Some are well off, some are considered not so well off, some have college, some have no college and two in fact did not graduate from high school. They are all considered middle class people. This book did not interview anyone who was considered "rich" or considered below poverty level.

The current ages of these nine people go from 67 (U.S. retirement age in 2028) to 98 years of age. These people's history to the age of 67 and beyond is thoroughly covered. Thus, one can see how they got to the retirement position they are now in. Then their lives in retirement are thoroughly covered along with their plans for the future. It includes their health, civic activities, and what they enjoy doing in retirement.

In this book you will find a prescription for a happy retirement-no matter what stage of life you are in. The cost of this book is about the same as three packs of cigarettes. Except that the information in this book could add many healthy and productive years to your retirement life.

Introduction

In 1930 the life expectancy average in the United States for all races and both sexes was 59.7.   In 2012 the life expectancy average for those born in the United States was 78.74 years.

If you graph the life expectancy growth from 1930 to 2010 and extend the graph to the year 2030, then this number extrapolates out on average to the age of 85 for children to be born in 2030.

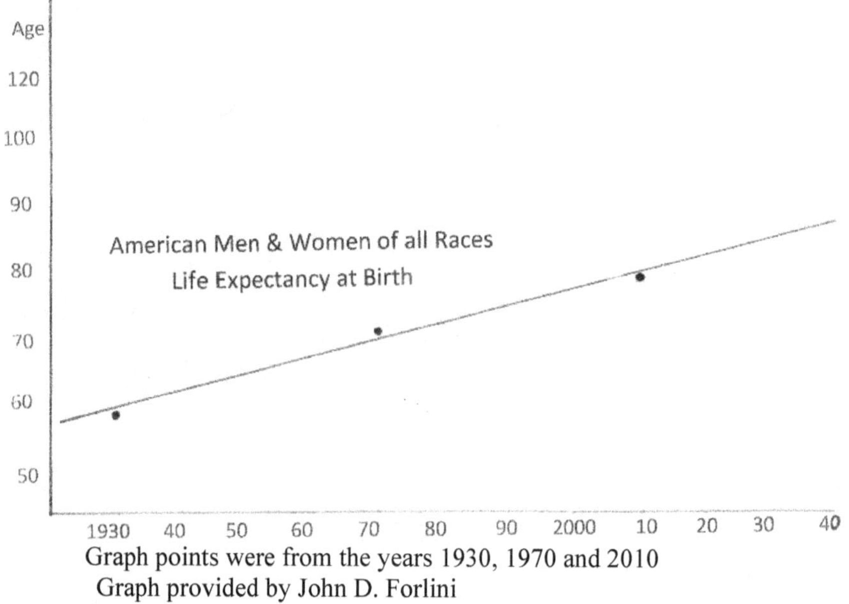

Graph points were from the years 1930, 1970 and 2010
Graph provided by John D. Forlini

So what does this mean? It means most people are going to have more time in retirement.   First, let's define retirement. Retirement is by definition in this book anyone 67 years of age or older.   In the United States it will be 2028 before this is officially the age of retirement.

At age 66 you can draw your social security benefit with no IRS negative impact to working income if you wish to continue working. This number was 65 for many years. In fact, 65 is still the age with which an individual can go on Medicare.

While retirement age is defined as 67 (in 2028), the census bureau statistics still use 65 as the age for reference points in their work. Their estimate of the number of 65 year olds or over in 2014 is 46.2 million out of a total U.S. population of 324 million or 14.25% of the population. This percentage is expected to increase each year.

The average individual American's retirement income is $18,000 per year. It should be pointed out that if a husband and wife both retire at retirement age of 66, the wife is entitled to half of her husband's social security. So if the husband has $20,000 per year of social security, then this household would receive $30,000 per year. Unless of course if the wife had a strong retirement of her own. Then the retirement income would be the combination of both retirements.

So if you are 67 or over, then you are retired—even if you are still working. There are those that have defined retirement as no longer working full time. But for this book it is anyone 67 or older.

If you are 67 or over, you have already been bombarded with retirement cons and programs to manage your money-assuming you have any. Or if you are like my wife and I, we have no money to truly invest. The census bureau lists $36,895 as the median income for households with someone 65 or older. That means half of these households are above this number and half are below.

At 74, we pay our bills, have a little left over for a modest yearly vacation, and dread the unexpected bill that may occur. We do have a plan that we believe will bring more security. And at the time of this writing I am now working part time and plan to continue for 3 more months or until our house sells.

By examining the ten people in this book who have either retired, are in process of retiring, or have been retired for several decades you can learn many valuable lessons and approaches to retirement. This book also incorporates recent writings and research on retirement to enhance the nine real life case histories.

While we have used 67 as the age of retirement, it is currently 66 and will not be 67 until those born in 1960 reach 67 or the year 2028.

In the biographies of these nine people, we will examine how they reached retirement and what they are doing in retirement and their plans for the future. A list of the people and their basic statistics are detailed below. Their names have been changed to give them anonymity.

The 9 Retirees in this Book

Name	Age	Education	Financial Strength	Health	Age Last Worked*	Plan Strength
Jeff	75	Masters	Moderate	Good	74.5	Good
Gloria	86	GED	Good	Fair	33	Poor
Roger	68	College	Moderate	Good	67	Good
Mary	94	High Sch.	Moderate	Failed	65	N.A.
Clete	98	8th Grade	Good	Poor	70	Good
Angie	79	High Sch.	Poor	Fair	60	Fair
Larry	76	Some Coll.	Excellent	Good	66	Good
Steve	84	MBA	Fair	Poor	66	Good
Lottie	73	College	Fair	Fair	65	Good

Each case history or biography starts with an overview of their basic statistics. It then relates their status at age 67. It then relates how they got to this point-their history to age 67. It provides a history of their life's work to age 67. It then goes on to describe in depth their financial, health, and entertainment activities at 67 and beyond. And then it tells of their future plans. The exact format for each of the nine case histories is as follows:

1. Overview
2. Situation at Age 67
3. History leading to Retirement
4. Retirement Years
   (67 and beyond)
5. Lifelong Monetary Plan
6. Plan for the Future

7. SWOT Analysis
   Strengths
   Weaknesses
   Opportunities
   Threats
8. Civic Activities
9. Regrets

10. Health Issues

At the end of each case history is a section entitled SWOT (Strengths, Weaknesses, Opportunities, and Threats). The SWOT analysis will show what each person's strengths are going forward with their lives along with their weaknesses, opportunities, and threats to their future in their remaining retirement years.

These case histories were chosen because they represent the breadth of experience that most retirees experience. Most chose their paths early on, but each was affected by the situations around them.

These nine case histories are a wealth of information for those now in retirement and for those who will someday reach the age of retirement. This book is written to give retirees and future retirees case histories that can provide insight to improve their own lives along with the recent literature in the final chapter.

You will find that some of these retirees truly prepared for retirement and some who did not give two cents to the possibility of retirement. I am one of those who never put a nickel away for retirement. But, I have a plan. And it's not to make money from this book, although it would be nice. This is my 14th book. While I get a royalty each month from one or more of my books, I only made $415.00 last year and about the same the year before. The average author of books only makes $150.00!

Chapter 1
(Jeffrey)

Name	Age	Education	Financial Strength	Health	Age Last Worked	Plan Strength
Jeff	75	Masters	Moderate	Good	74.5 yrs	Good

Overview

As can be seen by the chart above, Jeff is a 75 year old man. His level of education is at the Masters level (MBA) and his college degree was a major in chemistry. He minored in math and physics.

Jeff was at the extreme in that he never put a nickel away in savings. He did have a 401 K that fluctuated between $20,000 and $80,000, but he emptied it during his work years and during his early retirement years.

At age 70 he emptied his two 401k's to lower his monthly mortgage and take advantage of the low rates that existed at the time. He took both 401k's, one for $45,000 and one for $19,000 and was able to reduce his mortgage from $1,678 per month to $884 per month.

Jeff was fortunate that one of the many companies that he worked for had a pension plan. Jeff spent 13 years with this computer controls company until he was laid off at age 62. His retirement income from this company at 62 was $1,138 per month and started at the date he was laid off and will continue for the remainder of his life.

The computer controls company that Jeff worked for gave him a choice of $1,138 per month for just Jeff's longevity or $850 per month if his wife was put in the longevity mix. He and his wife chose the husband only option to have the greater income, gambling that Jeff would live as long as his wife. Jeff is 10 years older than his wife. At this point they have been collecting his retirement for 13 years.

As far as he knows, Jeff's health is good as shown in the chart. He takes no medicines other than a Synthroid supplement starting at age 66. He has never taken vitamins. He has run 5 times per week since he was in his early 20's; mostly 3 miles per day. However, at age 73 he had cut back on his distance, but still gets out there 5 times per week. He smoked unfiltered cigarettes from the age of 15 to age 26. Since age 26 he has been a strong opponent of anyone smoking.

Jeff is 5'9" and weighs (since high school) 145 pounds. In today's society Jeff is considered thin, although he believes he is right where someone his height should be. Jeff does not work out as such, but does 10 pushups and minor (5 minutes) calisthenics 6 days per week.

It might seem that Jeff should be financially well off, but he wasn't as you will learn. Jeff married right out of college 13 days after his 22nd birthday. This marriage lasted 13 years and bore 4 sons. It wasn't a bad marriage, but it lacked "something". Jeff did well financially because he worked obsessively. His wife was a stay at home mother and did a good job raising the kids. His wife was also going to school to obtain a Masters in psychology.

None of the companies that Jeff worked for during his first marriage had a retirement program and Jeff had very little in his bank accounts.

At the divorce, Jeff volunteered to give every bit of his assets to his wife and family, except a property in Gulf Shores, Alabama that had a high mortgage and provided a small rental income in the summer that paid half of the yearly mortgage. Jeff volunteered to pay child support until each child reached age 22.

Situation at Age 67

At 67 Jeff was "riding high". Financially he had three incomes coming in-His work income, his pension, and his social security as follows:

Work	$80,000 plus car allowance, which netted another $10,000
Pension	$13,656
Social S.	$28,000 Started at age 65 yrs. and 10 months.
Total	$131,656

At this point Jeff had been happily remarried for 31 years and this marriage produced a daughter, then 27 years of age and working on her PhD. Although Jeff had made more than $80,000 in his previous job, he was fortunate at his age to have this job. He had been working for this company for the past 4 years.

He was still not saving for retirement other than 10% of his income going to a 401k, which at this point totaled approximately $45,000. He had a balance of $18,000 in another 401k from his previous company.

Physically, Jeff was in great shape. He was still running and placing in first place in his age group in 5k races. He and his wife had a quiet social life, but they were happy. Much of their social life revolved around their daughter and people at work.

At work Jeff had just sold the largest single industrial order (4 Million dollars). This order turned out to have the highest profit of all orders over $500,000. Jeff was well liked at work and was well respected.

Jeff added a room and garage onto his house at age 67 so his daughter could move in and have her own space. It cost him $30,000. He did a good amount of the work himself. Jeff did most of the framing, he added a spiral staircase, did some of the wiring, and subcontracted the rest so this space would be ready in time for his daughter to move out of her apartment. She had been working, but decided to spend full time studying for a doctorate.

History leading to Retirement

Jeff was born in the Bronx borough of New York in the summer of 1942. He lived in a 6 story apartment building with his mother and father. The apartment was directly adjacent to the overhead El trestle subway system in New York.

Directly overhead two stories up, Jeff's Italian paternal grandparents lived in an identical apartment. His grandparents came from Italy right after they married. His grandfather was a brick layer.

Jeff and some of his friends would march off to PS 21 every day from Kindergarten through the 3rd grade. Most of the time one or another parent would accompany them at least through the second grade after which they were able to go by themselves.

The apartment that Jeff lived in had only one bedroom. It was a very small apartment with a living room and kitchen in addition to the single bedroom and bathroom. It was approximately 400 square feet overall.

When Jeff was six years old, he gained a brother. Jeff's father by this time was doing well as a salesman for an oil company. His job was to sell switching from burning coal for heat to burning oil in apartment buildings in New York.

When Jeff lived in the apartment building a coal truck would come and slide chutes into two ground level windows that allowed coal to flow into bins in the basement of the building. This coal was then periodically shoveled into a furnace that heated water into steam that was piped to radiators in each of the 6 stories of apartments. Jeff got into trouble playing in the coal chutes when he was younger.

For two years after the birth of Jeff's brother the family struggled with 4 people in the single bedroom. Fortunately, Jeff's father did well as a salesman and they moved across the Bronx line into Westchester where they built a two bedroom house.

Jeff's paternal grandfather and Jeff's grand uncle helped with the bricklaying and Jeff's maternal grandfather did the plaster work. His maternal grandfather had also come from Italy and was an excellent plasterer. Besides plastering walls he put up plaster figurines in churches. All 4 of Jeff's grandparents had come from Italy.

Jeff remembers the building of the house intimately. He would join his grandparents on the week-end while they were building the house. One of his most vivid memories came during the time when they were putting up the lathe that held the cement. This lathe and cement combination was then plastered over to make the final wall.

It was in January that they were putting up these walls. The house had no heat other than a barrel with some hot coal. His grandparents introduced him to hot coffee to keep him warm during the building of these plastered walls. He didn't care for the taste of the coffee, but it did warm him up. To this day he rarely drinks a cup of coffee. But when he does, it always brings back this memory.

In the Bronx Jeffrey was the leader of the pack of kids in his apartment building. He made up the games they played and the things that they did.

He wasn't a bad student nor was he particularly good. His report cards always said "Can do better". When he moved to Westchester and entered the 4th grade, he found that he was very far behind. The Bronx schools were not as advanced as the

Westchester schools. The school wanted to put Jeff back into the third grade to learn the multiplication tables and reading and vocabulary that he was behind in.

His mother wouldn't hear of it. She had a school teacher friend that agreed to tutor Jeff so he could remain in the 4th grade. Jeff did remain in the 4th grade and ended up doing reasonably well. By 6th grade Jeff found school boring and spent time "cutting up", but still managed to do reasonably well.

Jeff breezed through junior high and high school. His senior year of high school, Jeff obtained all B's and an A in physics. It was his best year for grades and for social life and for sports. He also received an award at the science fair.

He and his buddies put on a skit that landed them first prize in the school's talent contest. Jeff ran cross country and did well enough to receive a varsity letter. Jeff was also very active in the local fraternity that he and his buddies belonged to.

Jeff did get in trouble as the person responsible for holding a dance off school property where beer was had by Jeff and his friends. The town was upset enough over this incident that they established a teen set of rules called the "town pattern". Jeff could not be sanctioned by the school since it was an off-site event and not school related.

College was a different story for Jeff. He couldn't breeze through like he did in high school. He had to work hard and long for just passing grades. He majored in chemistry. He had not taken chemistry in high school, but he did well in his chemistry and math courses and thus minored in math and physics.

He had a desire to become a doctor because one of his friend's fathers was a doctor and Jeff felt that would be a real prestigious and rewarding career. He took the required zoology and comparative anatomy courses, but did poorly in both. He just did not like biology courses.

His senior year, he did apply to medical school, but only halfheartedly because he knew his grades were too low. Even straight A students were having difficulty getting accepted. He took an advanced organic chemistry course and did well and received a B. Chemistry ended up being the beginning of his career.

Jeff had decided on a major in chemistry for two reasons. First he liked chemistry and second it was a good fallback position if he did not get into medical school. Jeff's father died three months before Jeff finished college. His mother was well provided for, but there would be no money to help Jeff go on.

During college, Jeff worked as a waiter in a night club each summer. He also worked on a maintenance gang at the night club/resort. He was the only one on the crew that spoke English. He would work in maintenance from eight to five and then use the night club/resort's locker room to shower and get ready for the night of waiting on tables. These two jobs helped defray the cost of college for Jeff. Jeff also had a small scholarship.

Half way through his junior year, Jeff became engaged to his future wife. His wife was the same age, but was a year ahead in school. She graduated a year before Jeff and taught school during Jeff's senior year. Her teaching job was over 300 miles from Jeff's college.

Jeff gave her his 1955 Chevy that he had purchased and fixed up so she would have reliable transportation while teaching. For himself, Jeff found a1949 Mercury that he paid $60 for and used for transportation during his senior year. While it ran okay and lasted the whole year, it had too many things wrong for Jeff to keep it up and so he traded it for a 1956 used Buick convertible with a severe rust problem. It may have been rusty, but it ran like a dream.

Jeff was the first person on either side of his family tree to go to college. After graduation in June, Jeff went right to work back at the night club/resort. He immediately started looking for a job as a chemist while working at the night club. While he had three interviews at chemical plants, not one of these companies hired him. A fourth interview at a bakery in the Bronx netted Jeff his first industrial job.

In the middle of the summer, he married and it wasn't until September that he landed the bakery job. Jeff had enough money from his summer jobs to support himself and his wife in an apartment over a bar in Westchester. At his summer work he was paid in cash and Jeff bought everything he and his wife needed with cash. The bakery paid by check, but Jeff continued to pay cash for everything they purchased.

In March of the following year, Jeff was asked if he would transfer from the bakery to the company's newest acquisition, a large frozen foods company in Virginia. He readily accepted and he and his wife moved to Virginia. The company paid for his move. At this time his wife was pregnant with their first of 4 sons.

Jeff was a supervisor at the frozen foods company, but he still wasn't using his chemistry and he still wasn't working for a chemical plant. After a year at the frozen foods company, Jeff landed a job at a chemical plant in Virginia within a short driving distance from where he and his wife were living. It was now 1966, two years after graduating from college.

Jeff's wife was pregnant again. Their small apartment was going to be too small for their growing family. So Jeff decided they needed to purchase a house. In 1966 a house mortgage could be sold with the house. The new owner only had to keep up the mortgage payments after the mortgage and house were sold and transferred.

Jeff found a small three bedroom house for $16,500 with a mortgage payment of $105.00 per month. The only problem was that he had to come up with $2,500 for the down payment to assume the mortgage. He could scrape up $500, but that was it.

He decided to go to a bank and borrow the additional $2,000. The bank vice president that took his information told Jeffrey that he did not have enough assets or credit to obtain a loan. He explained in an arrogant manner that without having ever borrowed anything on time, that he had absolutely no credit for a loan. Jeff got the message as the bank vice president tore up the loan application.   He obviously felt that he had been wasting time on Jeff's application for a loan.

Jeff was a resourceful individual and devised a plan to get the $2,500. He went to a different bank and deposited $500.00. He then talked to the loan officer and explained that he wished to borrow $500.00 strictly to establish credit. He used his $500.00 deposit as "collateral". The bank loaned Jeff $500.00.

Jeff then took $500.00 and repeated this exercise at 4 more banks. The last bank was the first one he had gone to, but used a different loan officer than the original vice president. He now had the $2,500 he needed to buy the house. Jeff was naïve and didn't realize that what he had done was illegal. But he was now a bonafide home owner at age 24.

At the chemical plant, Jeff was making a good salary for his age. He was making $8,400 per year. In 1966 in Virginia this was very good pay. Shortly after the birth of his second son, the chemical plant had a massive explosion that killed the plant manager and severely burned one of the employees. Fortunately, Jeff had been working in a different building and was unhurt.

All of a sudden Jeff found himself in charge of the entire plant. It was a very small plant, but it was a major career move for Jeff. The owner of the plant was a brilliant scientist, but was dangerous in his method of operating the plant.

The owner had a laboratory at his house from which he developed the processes that the plant used to manufacture small batches of exotic chemicals. The owner never went to the plant because he had allergies that the chemicals affected. So he would give Jeff a rough idea of what to mix, heat, and distill. Some products were shipped out in liquid form and some were solid centrifuged products. Whenever Jeff went home, he smelled of chemicals and it took a great deal of scrubbing to come "clean".

The plant and chemicals were extremely dangerous. In 1966 in the hills of Virginia there were no quality standards. As a matter of fact after Jeff left the company a year later over a pay dispute, there were several more accidents and deaths. During Jeff's tenure there were no accidents or injuries. Years later the site became a "super fund site".

After leaving the plant, Jeff took a job in North Carolina with a 2,500 employee chemical plant that manufactured polyester. During the 3 months between jobs, Jeff made money driving a cab.

He was now on the way towards a long and profitable career in industry. He worked for this prestigious polyester company for 3.5 years. During this time, he made a name for himself by solving a major product flaw in one of the polyester products. He also wrote an article for a scientific journal for developing a gas chromatograph procedure to measure end product trace amounts of organic chemicals in the affluent at the plant.

Next Jeffrey took a position as a product development engineering group leader with one of the polyester plant end user companies located in Tennessee.

Jeffrey made a name for himself by saving the company hundreds of thousands of dollars with one of their products. He developed a procedure to reclaim products that would not operate properly at customer (paper mill) sites. Because of his success at this plant Jeff was placed on a fast track to upper management.

At this company, which had salesman located throughout North America and Europe, a senior management person had to have sales experience in the field. The average age of these salesmen was 50 years of age. Jeffrey was only 28.

So the company felt that before sending Jeff to the field as a salesman, he would have to spend at least 2 years in marketing. He was then promoted to manager of the proposal department. One of his functions was to sell products to the paper machine builders.

After a year successfully managing the proposal department, Jeff went up to the sales manager in early December and made a wager with him. There was a large potential order with a machine builder who wouldn't need product until the summer of the following year. This potential order was extremely competitive and would have been a major coup if it could be received by the end of the current fiscal year.

Knowing that the sales manager needed business by the end of December to make his "numbers" for the year, Jeff told the sales manager that he felt he could get this order by the end of December. The sales manager laughed at Jeff because he knew it was next to impossible. So Jeff bet him that if he did indeed get this order that the next available sales position would be his.

Jeff had become friendly with the project manager of the machine builder during the proposal stage. So with the bet with the sales manager accomplished, Jeff called his machine builder friend up and told him in a confidential manner that his (Jeff's) company would have a major price increase January 1.

To make a long story short, Jeff received a fax order from the machine builder on the last day of December. Jeff hand carried the order in to the sales manager and told him that his bags were packed and he was ready to move to California. Three days previously the California salesman had left the company leaving this opening for Jeff.

Jeff was excited, but unfortunately the General Manager of the company vetoed Jeff's move to California stating that this territory was too much of a "stretch" for Jeff. Jeff was upset and started looking for another job.

In February still working for this company as proposal manager, a friend of Jeff's met Jeff on Saturday at the office. This friend was also the manager of the southern sales district. He started off telling Jeff he had to shave his mustache off and purchase some conservative clothes. Jeff was floored because he couldn't see why his friend would care about these two items.

His friend smiled and said that salesmen in the south needed to be conservative looking to be able to make it. Jeff was being asked to take over the Alabama, Mississippi, western Florida, and southern Tennessee territory. So now he could really pack his bags and move to Mobile, Alabama.

The Mobile based salesman took Jeff around and introduced Jeff to some of the customers and paper mills in the region. The region had done poorly and never made its budgeted numbers. The salesman for this region admitted to Jeff that he really wasn't good at sales and therefore was taking a job in production at the corporate office in Tennessee.

Jeff took to sales as if he was a born salesman. He almost made the budgeted number of one million dollars. He only missed by fewer than fifty thousand. The next year when Jeff was in the job for the full year he made and exceeded his budget. The following year Jeff became the top worldwide corporate salesman and was the first to ever sell over $2 million in a year.

Jeff fell in love with Mobile and the Gulf Coast region. He enjoyed visiting customers in Panama City and Port St. Joe, Florida. He truly enjoyed being able to be at the beautiful beaches of the Gulf Coast and then spending time in the mountains of Tennessee.

During his fourth year of selling, he was offered a major promotion back to the home office in eastern Tennessee. But by this time Jeff had become a true southerner. He had purchased a lot on the water in Gulf Shores and built two summer cottages on this lot. By renting them out in the summer he could defray about 50% of the mortgage.

Jeffrey had changed. He no longer needed to climb the corporate ladder. He was happiest in sales. He enjoyed the freedom of determining his fate and he enjoyed all the people he worked with in the various paper mills. He knew his product well because he had been on the development side. He knew the when, where, who, and how of his job. And he was very successful.

He knew he could sell. So when the promotion came Jeffrey turned it down. He knew that this would hurt his career with his current company and so he looked for a job change that would allow him to stay in Mobile and still have some room for growth into a branch sales manager type position and still remain in Mobile.

Very quickly an electronics firm that made control gauging systems for paper machines and other parts of the plant grabbed him up. Jeffrey had no training in electronics, but he knew the paper mill business and knew the customers.

The electronics company put him in their 3 month training course in the home office in Ohio. He would spend 3 weeks in training and one week of each month in his territory. Jeff's training group of 3 salesmen was the first group to be introduced to computers. The company was taking its gauging equipment and connecting them to a computer and selling the package as a system with sophisticated controls.

Jeff enrolled himself in a computer course at South Alabama University in Mobile so he would be knowledgeable in computers. He obtained an A in the course. But more important he learned a significant amount to help him feel comfortable in his new job.

In his second year of sales with his new company, Jeff was number 2 in total sales for the company. The third year, Jeff was number one worldwide in a territory that the previous salesman said was "played out".

While Jeff should have been very comfortable in his life, he felt that his marriage was definitely missing something. He just felt that there had to be more than just working and coming home to a marriage without true love.

In discussing the situation with his wife, she agreed. They never had fights or disagreements, but there was no true love in the marriage. So they separated. Within a year they had both remarried.

Jeff agreed to a substantial monthly income for his family. He voluntarily agreed to pay this amount until the last child reached 22. He gave up the house, the car, and the bank account. He ended up with a sleeping bag and an old desk that he had fixed up.

Within a year Jeff found the love he was missing. He and his new wife would stay married and bear a wonderful daughter during their fourth year of marriage.

To be able to continue with his child support and have a home, Jeff had to sell one of his two cottages at Gulf Shores. Gulf Shores was trying to get owners to switch from septic tank to city water and sewage. Jeff offered to switch if the town would divide his property so he could sell one of the cottages.

The town agreed because they could then sell two meters instead of one.

He sold a cottage and agreed to hold a first mortgage for part of the sale. Interest rates at this time were 12-13% so Jeff obtained a 12% interest rate, which netted him $548 per month, which was almost half of his child support.

At this time Jeff and his wife purchased a small 17 foot Boston Whaler boat with a 60 horse power motor. Jeff loved to water ski. His wife would pull him on the ski's. They went to many lakes and enjoyed the boat.

While Jeff's love life had made a dramatic improvement, his business started to go sour. There were two factions in the company he worked for-the north and the south. The manager of the southern faction was beat out politically by the manager of the northern faction.

The manager of the southern faction left the company. The manager of the northern faction started firing branch managers in the southern region. Jeff's manager was the second one to go. Jeff knew it was only a matter of time before he would be let go as well.

Even though Jeff was about to be the top salesman for the year he was in, the new branch manager went after Jeff with a vengeance until they got into a heated argument. Jeff was fired the next week.

Within one week of being fired, Jeff was working for the competition. The previous company that fired Jeff refused to pay his earned commissions, which amounted to $35,000. Jeff took them to court and obtained a $50,000 judgment a year later.

Jeff was very successful with this new company, but with $40,000 left after paying his lawyer he decided to open a computer store in Mobile. He resigned from the company he was working for. They offered him a branch manager's job if he stayed, but Jeff wanted to be able to stay at home and not travel so much.

He borrowed $30,000 and opened up a store. At this time, 1981, personal computers were still a novelty. During the year of staying at home managing the store, Jeff and his wife had a baby girl. While he was financially surviving at best with his store, he knew that this was not for him. After slightly over a year, he sold his business at a loss, but he was out from under any obligations for lease, etc.

Jeff's wife was from Pensacola. She wanted to be closer to family now that she had a baby. So Jeff took several trips to Pensacola to find a job. He was quite lucky to quickly (within a month) find a job with a controls integrator in Pensacola.

It was a relatively small company, but with a $400.00 monthly tax free car allowance on top of a salary of $40,000 he was able to do okay. They sold their house in Mobile and moved to Pensacola. Jeff commuted until the house sold.

In Pensacola, they built a modest house that suited their needs. With child support partially offset by the first mortgage on the cottage they were able to get by for a while. But, eventually (within 5 years) they had to sell the second cottage to keep going. Eventually the mortgage holder on the first cottage paid off the $35,000 balance left on the mortgage. This helped for a considerable while.

Jeff had worked his way up to sales manager of the controls company. He was now making $53,000 per year. However, after two years of sales manager Jeff hired a salesman that ended up causing Jeff to resign from the company.

Within a week Jeff was working for a prestigious maker of controls and computer systems for all industries worldwide. He obtained a considerable raise in making this change. More important, this new company had a lucrative pension plan. After 13 years with this company, Jeff was laid off as part of a major downsizing,   but, at this time, Jeff was 62 and able to collect this pension at $1,138.00 per month.

He was no longer paying child support because his children by his first marriage were in their twenties, thirties, and his oldest was now 40. He no longer had a relationship with his sons. His ex-wife and her husband had moved the boys away within two years of the divorce and she made seeing his children a difficult and heart wrenching proposition for everyone.

Jeff's daughter had elected to go to a very expensive private college out of state. Jeff covered all tuition, living, and expenses for this 4 year school.

When Jeff was laid off at 62, he had just sold his house and with the profit he made, he paid off $100,000 on a note for a piece of land on the water that he and his wife were planning to build a house on. Jeff had no capital left and had to scramble with odd sales jobs to keep up the duplex apartment rent and living expenses.

Jeff and his wife were renting a duplex directly on the bay in Pensacola. It had a beautiful view, but unfortunately a major hurricane eleven months into the rental devastated this unit. Jeff and his wife had no place to live.

So they got in their car and had just enough gas to reach the first open gas station still in operation after the devastating hurricane. From there they made it to Birmingham. Jeff had enough Marriott rewards to stay 12 nights free in a Marriott Town Place Suites that came complete with a kitchenette.

It took ten days where Jeff's duplex was located before Jeff was able to get back in to his unit in Pensacola. Jeff and his wife rented a large U-Haul and returned to Pensacola to pick up whatever they could in the way of their remaining furniture.

Water had filled up the bottom two floors where the garage, storage, and master bedroom were located. The living room furniture on the third floor was unharmed. Their bed on the first floor was still saturated with water and had to be left.

They were able to take the wooden bedroom furniture after drying it off. The mirror on the dresser was broken and part of the mirror had been carried out to sea. Jeff had a mirror cut to size and was able to restore the dresser to its original look.

They had just enough room in the U-Haul truck and a U-Haul connected to their van to transport their belongings. By this time they had signed on an apartment in Birmingham and were to have a new bed delivered the next day after they arrived with their U-Hauls.

For 4 months in Birmingham Jeff sold health insurance and mortgages. He then landed a job with a controls integrator similar to the one he had worked with in his earlier career in Pensacola. Jeff contacted them directly and it just so happened they were looking for a sales engineer. He lucked out again. So at the age of 63 Jeff was back working full time in the industry he had worked in most of his career.

Retirement Years (Beyond 67)

As mentioned earlier, Jeff was doing very well with this controls integrator at age 67. He continued to do well, but the company changed while Jeff was out selling his heart out. He had received an excellent performance review in January of his last year with the company. The company reorganized and Jeff no longer worked directly for the president.

Just before his 69th birthday, Jeff was laid off even though he had just received this excellent performance review from the president of the company.

He was the first of three sales people laid off at or around age 69. They could have gotten together to initiate an age discrimination suit and probably won. But Jeff went to work with a competitor, and didn't have any inclination to work with lawyers.

The same week that Jeff turned 70, he decided to retire from industry and write books. Although he barely worked a full year for this latest controls integrator, he just felt it was time to leave.

One month prior to turning 70, Jeffrey refinanced his house. He was paying $1,684.35 per month for his mortgage. Jeff decided to use his entire 401k to lower his amount mortgaged and refinance the balance.

The new rate that he obtained for a 30 year fixed mortgage was 3.35% and coupled with the proceeds from his 401k lowered his monthly to 888.65 per month. The difference then was ($1,684.35 - $888.65) which was $795.70 per month or $9,548.40 annually. Although the stock market has done well, in 5 years Jeffrey saved $47,742 which was more than he would have made if he had left the stocks in his 401k and- it was risk free and tax free.

For the next 3 years, Jeff wrote and published over 10 books. He received royalties each and every month, but they were only between $80 and $100 dollars per month.

Right after Jeff turned 73 his daughter announced that she was to be married the end of October. Jeff had to borrow the money for the wedding by obtaining a line of credit for $25,000. He decided to go back to work to pay off the line of credit. He told everyone that he was bored with writing and missed the industrial market, which was true. He also needed to pay off the line of credit.

So for the next 14 months Jeff was back working for a controls integrator. This would be the fourth control's engineering and construction firm that he worked for. After 14 months he had finally decided to leave industry all together. He was now 74 and 1/2 years of age. He had done well with this last controls integrator, but decided that he had had enough.

He had paid off his debts and had $9,000 in his first real savings account. The only problem was that in doing his income tax he had a $13,000 combined federal and state income tax. So he was still $4,000 in the hole. But, if he could sell his Model A for $15,000 he would be back in the black. He and his wife also had their house for sale by owner. If they got their price of $389,000, this would leave them with $209,000 in cash.

Lifelong Monetary Plan

While it may seem that Jeff did not have a true monetary plan, since he never saved any money, he did in fact have a life's plan. He did not invest directly in stocks or bonds. The only stocks and bonds that he invested in were through his 401k.

What Jeff decided early on was that he would rather enjoy his investments rather than have paper like stocks and bonds. So his savings were in the form of real estate. Taxation, especially on private homes and even rentals was nothing compared to other investments.

In all, Jeffrey over the years had 7 nice personal homes, 2 rental properties, and 2 rental cottages on the water at Gulf Shores. With the exception of the house that his first wife received upon divorce, Jeff made a profit on each house. In all, he made approximately $266,000 virtually tax free. Of this he still has a piece of land on the water in Pensacola that is paid for. The worth of this property is around $150,000. When he sells his current house he should walk away with over $200,000 tax free.

At age 74 Jeffrey had his first full year without spending on his 5 children. His child support for his first four children was completed when he was 56. Jeffrey never begrudged his expenditures on children and in fact was proud that he was able to do it. He was proud that they all had college and extra proud that several had advanced degrees and one even obtained a doctorate.

Jeff tried going into business three times. Once during the beginning of the 1980's he opened a computer store. He sold it slightly after a year. Each time he tried to go into business it was clear he could make more money in industrial sales working for a company already doing business.

Plan for the Future

Jeff's and his wife's plan for the immediate future is to sell their house, take $175,000 out of the approximately $210,000 equity and build a place on their water lot in Pensacola. This would leave approximately $20,000-35,000 in cash depending on whether they sold their Model A and how much it cost to move.

Jeff's retirement income is $53,200 per year and barely covers yearly expenses. Jeff plans to sell real estate when they move to Pensacola to supplement the $53,200. He would only have to make $17,000-$20,000 per year to live very comfortably. Even though he plans to build his house for cash, he will take out a mortgage of $100,000 leaving a monthly slightly over $400. He feels that he could do that and live leisurely taking several vacations each year.

SWOT Analysis

Strengths:

Jeff's main strength is his health and stable life style. He takes no medicines and at 74½ he has a decent retirement income. He also has a reasonable plan for the future. He believes that he can build a house for $175,000 and after two years sell it for $600,000 with no taxation on the profit.

He would then build a second house in the same development on the water. There are two lots currently for sale on the water in this development. Jeff is an excellent carpenter and has built numerous garages, Florida rooms and other additions to his homes. He can build this house with a substantial amount of subcontracting. In the past, he built several two story units. He learned to make stairs and developed many other building skills.

As mentioned, Jeff plans to take a $100,000 mortgage at roughly $450 per month, thereby leaving him with $120,000-135,000 in cash. He has always been cash poor and while this is not a fortune, it at least balances his portfolio.

Based on market conditions he may take part of this and diversify into stocks and bonds with extremely low risk. He has not made any decisions on this aspect as of yet. He also has his eye on a rental property in a subdivision in Pensacola that he once lived in. He probably won't purchase a rental until he lives in his Pensacola property for two years and then sells it at a good profit to build a second home. At any rate he plans to have good vacations each year even possibly spending as much as $6,000.

Weaknesses:

Jeff does not have a balanced portfolio at this time, although his plans are to balance it after he sells his home. All of his assets are in real estate. He has no cash and in fact has a $4,000 income tax deficit that he will carry on his Master Card at zero interest. He has not yet sold either his house or his Model A. He has never sold real estate and expects there will be a learning curve. His yearly income of $53,000 is just marginal. Inflation will make it tighter as time goes on.

Opportunities:

Jeff obtained his real estate license at age 69 just prior to full employment with the integrator company that he was with prior to leaving and writing books. This license has been on inactive status since he obtained it. Jeff's plan is to convert this Alabama license to a Florida license with a simple Florida test related to Florida rules. Alabama and Florida have a reciprocal agreement so Jeff does not have to go through the main testing.

Jeff's main opportunity is the sale of his home and his Model A. He would have approximately $220,000 with these two sales. If Jeff is correct in his estimates about building and selling the house he builds on the water, then he has an opportunity to double his assets in two years. And then repeat the process. He would then have a house on the water with no mortgage and $250,000 in cash. He could take reasonable vacations for many years with this money. At $6,000 per year he could vacation lavishly for 25 years bringing him to the ripe age of 100.

His income from real estate could make this even higher. If he has enough cash, he could purchase a rental property to increase his yearly income. He needs to be careful and not have all his assets in real estate.

This past year was the first time since Jeff and his wife were married that they had no outgo for children. He has a $4,000 debt incurred from income taxes and his daughter's wedding that he carries on his Master Card. He and his wife have a 6 month plan to pay it off.

Threats:

Jeff's age is a threat. He is embarking on a new life at age 75.
Will he have the energy and health to do it? He or his wife could
become seriously ill. The housing market could change. It
could take a long time to sell his existing home and Model A.

Rental cost in Pensacola while Jeff is building could be a
drain on their $53,000 yearly income. Jeff may not be able to
sell real estate as readily as he thinks.

Civic Activities

Jeffrey is not currently involved in any civic activities.
However, throughout his life Jeffrey has given back by helping
others. Most recently he had signed up with a civic organization
called Vitas. At Vitas Jeffrey gave presentations on the 1930's
to nursing homes.

Prior to this Jeffrey was involved with home building for the
needy. Jeffrey taught Sunday school to 7th and 8th graders.
Jeffrey always stopped to help stranded motorists. His
mechanical expertise enabled him to get them moving again.

In both of his marriages, Jeffrey was the sole bread winner so
that his wives could do civic and volunteer work. Both wives
did a good deal of both.

Regrets

Everyone can look back in their life and enumerate regrets.
Jeff has only three major regrets. By far his greatest regret is
that he did not and does not have a relationship with his sons.
Jeff feels that it was an impossible situation, yet he still feels that
there must have been something he could have done.

All of his boys have done well in life. They each made it
through college and two have a Master's in Business and one a
doctorate. Jeffrey is proud of them and is grateful that they have
done well. He just wishes he could have been part of their lives
after the divorce.

He regrets ever having smoked. He smoked from the age of
15 to the age of 27. He has been plagued with hoarseness of
voice for the last several years. He believes it is from acid reflux
compounded by his years of smoking. He can control it, but it

meant giving up running, which he enjoyed immensely. He still goes out each day and walks what he used to run.

His third regret is the college that he chose. He chose it because it had the lowest tuition, he had a scholarship in New York State, and this college had a good reputation.

He regrets going to college in the Snow Belt south of Buffalo because of the extreme cold and snow. But, most of all he regrets going to such a small school. Jeff didn't join a fraternity. What he didn't realize was that fraternities had each professor's previous year's tests. This gave Jeff's class mates a distinct advantage. Jeff believes that had he not smoked and had he gone to a different college that his grades would have been significantly higher. He later proved this with his Master's degree.

Health Issues

Jeffrey doesn't really have any serious health issues. He does not take medicines, except for a thyroid supplement (50 Micrograms of Synthroid six times per week).

He had been running up until he was 74 ½. He stopped (temporarily) because of hoarseness and slight pain in his vocal chords. He attributes this to his running and to his earlier years of smoking. He feels that running churns up the acid in his stomach and causes acid reflux, which irritates his vocal chords. So for now instead of running 15 miles per week, he is walking this same distance and a little more.

He has also eliminated milk, desserts (he ate dessert at least once per day and many times 2 times per day), and chocolate. He had problems with hoarseness off and on most of his married life. So he had already given up coke, coffee, and mayonnaise.

In the past, if he was careful with his eating, the hoarseness would go away. Then he could gradually add back some of the foods that he had eliminated. This time it is taking longer to go away. This is the first time he has given up running to eliminate the hoarseness.

Chapter 2
(Gloria)

Name	Age	Education	Financial Strength	Health	Age Last Worked	Plan Strength
Gloria	86	GED	Good	Fair	33	Good

Overview

As can be seen by the chart above, Gloria is an 86 year old woman. She did not graduate with her high school class, but obtained a GED later in her 30's.

Gloria and her second husband were both way past frugal. At night they would go to the bathroom and not flush until the morning to save money on water. They were to the furthest right on the frugality scale.

Gloria is 5'5" and weighs approximately 128 pounds. She takes many medicines including Coumadin, blood pressure medicine, cholesterol medicine, and a variety of other drugs and vitamins and minerals.

Gloria grew up in farm country in western north Florida about 40 miles from Tallahassee almost on the Georgia border.

She grew up on an 80 acre farm. Her father was a poor farmer who also did carpentry work from time to time. He fought in WW II in France and Germany. He was a cook in the army. Her mother worked in a cigar factory until the war was over. Growing up on the farm, Gloria's main job was to look after her brothers and sisters.

Between her first husband and her second husband, Gloria worked several different jobs. She married her second husband when she was 33. From then on she was a stay at home person. For one of the four years between marriages Gloria parked her two children with her mother on the family farm. It was the best time for her children. They still remember the wonderful way their grandmother cared for them.

Gloria does no physical activities. She never went for walks or exercised. At 86 she still drives a car, but very slowly and cautiously.

Gloria is living on her and her dead husband's pension and social security. She has a large bank account and stocks and bonds of approximately $800,000. All of her money came from her second husband. He had a secure job at the naval base in aircraft maintenance.

What made them well off was an inheritance that her second husband (Fred) obtained from an uncle. The uncle had land that Fred inherited and sold to Disney World. Fred never touched the money. He simply invested it and he and Gloria lived off his salary from his foreman's job at the navy base. Some of his investment did pay dividends and still does.

Gloria has alienated virtually her whole family. She has told them all they are nothings and doesn't want them to come to her home. She basically sits in her house. She still drives and therefore does her shopping. She gets her hair done once per week. She insists that her children have been stealing from her as do some of her siblings. This is not the case at all. She claims to anyone that will listen that they have stolen screw drivers, drills, etc.

Situation at Age 67

At age 67 Gloria was as secure as an individual could be, at least financially. Her husband Fred was now retired. He retired early on a pension from his job at the naval air station. He received approximately $28,000 per year. Gloria received a social security check each month for $300.

In addition, they received approximately $15,000 in dividends. What made them both so secure wasn't their combined income of $48,400, but their lack of significant outgo.

Their home was paid for, their taxes were barely $1,000 per year and they had no extravagances. In their entire married life, they took only 4 vacations. They took several motor trips to Branson, Missouri, and they went with Gloria's sister's family to North Carolina for a week. They ate out once per week at frugal restaurants like Cracker Barrel.

Gloria made Fred's life miserable by always making up possible transgressions that Fred did not commit. No arguing on his part would convince her that he was innocent. And he was innocent every time. She watched Fred like a hawk. He virtually never went anywhere without her being along.

She would accuse him of secretly calling some of his relatives or worse. She would get it into her head that he had done something and no matter what proof she was shown she would still insist it was true. His life was miserable. Not that he was anywhere near perfect.

He was an extremely cold individual and a miser as well. In this both Gloria and Fred were in step. They were both misers. Although, Gloria was worse than Fred. Years before she was 67, she would even hold back lunch money from her kids. Her youngest daughter sold pecans and Gloria would take some of her change for her own purposes and never pay her daughter back.

At 67, they had sold their first house, the one that Gloria had purchased for $5,000. They sold it to Gloria's oldest daughter for $30,000 to be paid monthly at $150 per month with no interest until it was paid for. Fred and Gloria purchased a new house for $56,000 and paid cash. Thus, at age 67 Gloria had no mortgage and more income than outgo. Their approximate income was as follows:

```
Pension--  $28,000
Social S.   $ 3,600
Dividends  $15,000
Mortgage   $ 1,800 Daughters payments
   Total   $ 48,400
```

History leading to Retirement

As mentioned, Gloria was not a very good student. For her last two years of high school she went to school in Tallahassee. She stayed with an Aunt.

Gloria dropped out in her senior year without getting her diploma. She soon married Joseph. Joseph had a good job laying tile in houses, motels, and other buildings. He had been working since he was 14. His family forged a birth certificate so he could join the service when he was 15. All his money went to his family.

When Joseph and Gloria married, Joseph still sent money home to his family. Joseph and Gloria moved to Pensacola and Gloria quickly put an end to Joseph sending money to his family.

Shortly after they were married, Joseph would drink until he was totally wasted. He would make good money and then "lay out" drunk for a period of time. When he was drunk and sometimes when he was sober he would physically abuse Gloria.

Somehow this dragged on through the addition of two girl children.

Both girl children vividly remember their parents fighting. The father was actually good to the girls especially when he was sober and even when he was drunk. He took them to the beach. He bought them bicycles. However, by the time the girls were 7 and 8 their father was mostly gone and did not support them.

When the girls were 5 and 6 they went to live with Gloria's parents near Tallahassee for a full year. During this time, Gloria found several jobs and got on her feet. Her husband was totally gone by the time the girls returned to Pensacola.

Gloria had to work to support the family. She didn't have a high school diploma, but Pensacola was a good town to work in at this time and so she managed to get some decent jobs. She worked for the main industrial plant (Chemstrand) and then she worked in grocery stores and as a waitress at a night club. During this time she obtained her GED.

When Gloria's two girl children were growing up, Gloria treated them like 4th class citizens. Even after she was married to her second husband and had a solid income, she still deprived her children. She virtually did not buy them clothes. They had to work at babysitting to purchase patterns and material to make their own clothes.

Before she married her second husband, she and the girls moved from apartment to apartment. Sometimes they were put out on the street for lack of payment. By the time they were 8 and 9, their mother was making enough to start a small savings. She managed to save her tips from the night club. The girls remember this time as their best part of childhood.

The girls did all the shopping and did the cooking and cleaning. Gloria would go out with her girlfriends and didn't think much about her daughters during their pre-teens. They went to school without food many times. There was no money for lunches.

When the youngest girl was 11, Gloria purchased a house that was a mess, but it was livable. She paid $5,000 for a mortgage with little to no money down. The youngest girl sold pecans for spending money to buy material to make her clothes.

By the time the youngest girl, Terry, was 12, Gloria married Fred, her second husband. Fred was extremely cold to the two daughters, but he provided food and spent some money fixing up

Gloria's house. He added air conditioning and other minor items.

Fred would go to work at 6:00 A.M. and return at dinner time. He would monopolize the little TV and the girls had to be in bed by 9:00 A.M. Neither Fred nor Gloria spent any time with the two girls. They knew nothing of their homework. The two girls spent most of their time in their tiny rooms.

All of her life Gloria was self-centered and extremely stingy. Even though her husband brought home a good income, Gloria continued to be stingy. Her youngest learned to use a sewing machine that she bought herself with money she made working. She did a great deal of baby sitting and sold pecans that she picked and found on the ground. She would bag them into small units and sell them door to door.

Right after the oldest girl Rhonda graduated from high school, she went off by bus to visit her father in North Carolina. He was supposedly working a job there. What she was really doing was meeting her boyfriend there to get married. He was at Camp Lejeune in basic training.

When Gloria and Fred found out what Rhonda had done they were furious. They took it out on the youngest girl blaming her for not telling them what her older sister was planning to do. However, the youngest daughter did not have any idea what Rhonda was up to. She learned of it at the same time as Gloria.

Nothing that Terry could say or do would convince Gloria or Fred that she had no idea that Rhonda was going to elope. This wasn't the first time that no matter what Terry said, she wasn't believed.

Terry was a really good kid, but one day Gloria read that there were drugs in Terry's high school. So one afternoon when Terry returned home from high school, Gloria berated her for taking drugs. Terry would never take drugs even if she had the money, which she certainly didn't. Gloria told Terry that she knew that she was taking drugs and demanded the names of the other students. It was pure crazy on Gloria's part, but not unusual behavior for Gloria.

This wasn't the first or last time that Gloria would be unreasonably cruel to her daughter. She once accused Terry of rubbing against Fred. This was so absurd that it was ludicrous.

As soon as the youngest daughter graduated from high school she started looking for full time employment. During high school she had worked at a dentist's office as a receptionist.

Terry walked along the downtown area of Pensacola. She would go into each store looking for employment. She lucked out and found a job at a large furniture store in the downtown area. She worked in clerical positions and when the furniture company built a second store in the North end of Pensacola, she was transferred to the new store.

Gloria took Terry to work in the mornings and Terry usually got a ride home from someone at work. Terry saved her money and purchased a used car so she could get back and forth to work. Gloria never helped Terry other than the occasional morning rides to work. Terry was on her own. She was forced to pay Gloria part of her earnings for living at the house and transporting her to work.

Shortly after purchasing her own car, Terry found an apartment and moved out. Gloria was furious because she no longer had Terry's rent money. Gloria refused to go see her daughter's new apartment because she felt slighted by her daughter's moving out.

Gloria never participated in any social or civic organizations. She got up, made breakfast, packed a lunch, and saw Fred off to work. That was her life. She never went out of her way to help anyone including her family. Whenever anything happened it was how this would affect Gloria, not how it would affect those involved. Gloria's household was never a happy household.

When Terry was about 23, Gloria had to have a hysterectomy. Fred asked Terry if she would stay at their house and look after everything while Gloria was recuperating. Terry dutifully stayed with Fred and Gloria. She took care of the house and meals.

Gloria's husband Fred asked Terry if her mother was paying Terry's car payments as compensation for staying during the recuperation from the hysterectomy. He had told Gloria to pay Terry. So Terry received no compensation for her dutiful assistance.

Almost every day Gloria would accuse Terry of having secret conversations about her with Fred. It was ridiculous. Terry stood it for a month and then had to leave to get away from Gloria's insane accusations.

When Terry was 26 she married the love of her life, John. He was a successful businessman. After 5 years of marriage they built a house in Pensacola, just slightly after Gloria and Fred built theirs. As a matter of fact when Gloria decided to have a house warming for her and Fred's house, Terry's house was almost finished.

Many guests were invited to Gloria's home for the house warming, mostly aunts and uncles from Tallahassee. Terry and Rhonda and their husbands went as well. Gloria asked Terry to cater the event. It was costly. Gloria never paid anything for the event and never thanked Terry for handling the whole thing.

As a matter of fact, Gloria accused Terry of "showing off". One of the aunts who learned that John and Terry were also building a house wanted to go over to see it.

Terry didn't want to show it and said that the house wasn't complete yet.   However, the whole group travelled over there. While the house wasn't finished, it was a beautiful two story home. One of the aunts made the comment, "My, this house just dwarf's Gloria's house".

It was tactless, but not Terry's fault. Terry was afraid one of the aunts would say something like that and therefore didn't want to show her house. She also knew that Gloria would get onto her about it. Terry just couldn't win. It was like that with Gloria all of Terry's life. No matter what she did it wasn't enough. Worse, Gloria would accuse Terry of all kinds of ridiculous things. She again accused not only Terry, but her whole family of being on drugs.

John and Terry had a daughter that was a high achiever. Whenever their daughter, Melisa had an event like a recital, soccer game, or graduations Terry would invite Gloria. Gloria never went. Gloria was just not interested in her grandchild.

When Terry's daughter was 8 years old, Terry had the traditional Thanksgiving Turkey meal for the family at her house as she had several times in the past. Gloria and Fred and Rhonda and her husband and three children were in attendance as well. Terry always outdid herself with a great prepared meal with all the trimmings and desserts, etc.   The house was always immaculate.

The next day, Gloria told Terry that she wasn't comfortable in Terry's house. In addition, Terry's sister and husband left early to go to the dog track. Terry was understandably upset, but used to her mother's mean streak. John suggested that from now on they would go to Pigeon Forge and enjoy Thanksgiving with just the three of them.

They did from then on and enjoyed each Thanksgiving immensely. To this day, Pigeon Forge is special to Melisa and it is special to John and Terry as well. They go there every year.

Gloria's husband retired early as mentioned. He worked in the yard some, but mostly sat in his recliner and watched television all day long. Gloria piddled around the house and did some work in the yard. They went out to eat every Saturday night. That's it. That's how they lived.

Retirement Years (Beyond 67)

Gloria and Fred continued to live the same for the next 20 years. They did go to Branson, Missouri twice and they went twice to North Carolina with Gloria's sister and husband. But otherwise they did nothing. They were invited to visit for Thanksgiving and Christmas at Gloria's older daughter's house. They would occasionally visit Gloria's younger sister who also lived in Pensacola for a period of time until the younger sister and her husband moved to Fairhope, Alabama.

Gloria and Fred continued to build up their savings account because they spent so little on themselves. They certainly never spent anything on anyone else.

When Gloria was 80, Fred started showing signs of dementia and this went into full blown Alzheimer's by the time Gloria was 83. Fred refused to bathe and just sat and would not talk by the time Gloria was 84. Fred died in the hospital when Gloria was 85 and Fred was 89.

At 85 Gloria was still physically able to drive. Her eldest daughter had helped Gloria with the funeral arrangements for Fred. She and her husband also helped with cutting the grass and other chores. Whenever they had an activity at their house like a birthday for children or grandchildren, Gloria was always invited.

Yet Gloria decided that her eldest daughter and her husband were stealing from her. She accused them of stealing screwdrivers, drills, switching tires, and rifling through her papers. None of these tales were true, yet Gloria insisted on telling anyone that would listen that her daughter and especially Rhonda's husband was a thief.

Shortly after this started Gloria came down with shingles. Her youngest daughter and her husband came to Pensacola and took Gloria back to their home in Birmingham. Her daughter bathed her and put ointment on her each day. For 4 months Gloria was well cared for.

Just as Gloria was almost totally recovered, her daughter caught her listening in on a phone conversation. When her daughter caught her, Gloria said that she always felt her daughters were nothing and still thought they were just nothing. Naturally her daughter and her husband returned Gloria to her home in Pensacola.

Gloria persisted in telling everyone that now both daughters and one of her brothers had been stealing from her. She would call relatives up on the phone and complain that people were stealing from her. She threatened her oldest daughter by calling her up and telling her she had a gun in the house and would use it on anyone coming in the house to steel. The youngest daughter still periodically calls to check and make sure Gloria is alright.

At the age of 86 Gloria still drives. She goes to a beauty shop each week, yet spends very little money. She eats sparingly with TV dinners, one or two outside meals, and frugal store bought food on a weekly basis. She doesn't watch television and does not own a computer. She takes good care of herself, but spends very little.

She just mainly sits and occasionally talks on the phone to anyone in the family that will still listen to her. However, most of the family is sick and tired of Gloria's rants about everyone.

She now has a yard man to care for the grass cutting and other odd chores. Her income from her husband's pension and her own social security covers her needs. Plus she has a good bank account and dividends from stocks and bonds.

She shows no signs of Dementia. She will never discuss her financial situation with anyone, but this is what is known. She refuses to make out a will. If she did she said she would give everything to the Alzheimer's foundation. This is Gloria and Gloria's retirement as she approaches her 87th birthday.

Plan for the Future

Gloria does not have a fixed plan for the future. She is just going to keep living every day and do what she has always done. She will take her medicines, see her doctors, and go to the beauty shop each week. She will guard her possessions with her life.

SWOT Analysis

Strengths:

Gloria's main strength is that Fred has left her financially well off. She has no mortgage and has a very low house tax. Her car is in good shape. Her income exceeds her outgo and she has a strong capital reserve. As long as she keeps taking her medicines she should live another 6 to 10 years or more. This is based on the long lives of her aunts.

Weaknesses:

Gloria has no life. She is financially sound, but is limited in her mental capacity to do anything but exist. She does absolutely no physical exercise. This will eventually lead to her body shutting down. Although she shows no signs of Alzheimer's, her mental condition is not strong and this could lead to problems down the road. Plus her paranoia, which she has had all her life seems to be getting worse.

Opportunities:

Gloria has no real opportunities. She has alienated her daughters and some of her brothers and sisters. She lives alone and has virtually few real friends.

Threats:

Gloria's biggest threat comes from living alone with virtually no one other than her youngest daughter checking up on her by phone once per week. She refuses to wear a medical alert aid. She rarely uses her hearing aid. Both could lead to medical problems that would take days to come to anyone's attention.

Regrets

It is not known if Gloria has any specific regrets. She definitely enjoyed having people believe her lies about others and probably regrets that no one will take her lies seriously anymore. She had always expected and demanded that everything revolve around her. Virtually no one fools with her anymore and this has to be a major regret.

Chapter 3
(Roger)

Name	Age	Education	Financial Strength	Health	Age Last Worked	Plan Strength
Roger	68	Elect. Eng	Moderate	Good	67 yrs	Good

Overview

As can be seen by the chart above, Roger is a 68 year old male in good physical shape. He worked until he was 67 and then retired. His retirement included part time work with the company that he retired from. He is also looking for additional part time work in the marketing communications and content development arena.

Roger is married with one 35 year old son that is physically and intellectually disabled. This requires Roger and his wife of 39 years to be constant caregivers. They do this willingly and this shows the strong character of both Roger and his wife.

At the time of his retirement at 67 Roger was making good money from his job plus he had a solid 401k. Roger did not have any debts because he paid everything on time other than his mortgage related debt. His mortgage debt amounted to $800.00/month.

Roger is 5'7" and weighs 175. He does take blood pressure medicine and he does have a stent that was put in in 2005. Generally, he is in good physical shape and is working to get his weight down to 165. Roger does some physical exercise. He walks multiple times per week.

Roger is college educated and has worked in marketing at his most recent controls engineering company and worked in marketing with prior companies. He let his credit cards get ahead of him at one time years ago and thus does not use regular credit cards anymore. He does have a debit card.

Roger's wife has a small arts and crafts business that barely breaks even each year. She does this as a creative outlet more than as a money maker.

Not one of the companies that Roger worked for had a pension plan. Thus his retirement must rely totally on social security and an annuity recently purchased from his 401(k) rollover that brings in $270 per month. Roger's part time work with his former company plus any additional work that Roger can obtain are the only supplements to his social security.

Roger believes that if he can supplement his social security with approximately $1,000 per month that he can survive with his current needs. He has to get through the next year with his wife's health insurance costs until she turns 65 and Medicare kicks in. Roger is counting on Medicare/Medicaid to continue to help with his son's medical costs as well.

Situation at Age 67

At 67 Roger was at the top of his career, but in a few months he would retire. Financially, Roger had two incomes now; His work income and his social security. His wife was not yet signed up for social security. His yearly income at 67 and his income at retirement at 68 are as follows:

	Age 67		Age 68
Social Security--	$ 31,200	Soon to be	$ 46,800
Work income	$ 90,000	Soon to be	$ 12,000 for part time
Annuity	$ 00,000	Soon to be	$ 3,240
Totals	$ 121,200		$ 62,040

When Roger left his full time job, his income dropped virtually to almost half. Roger believes that he can live adequately with his new income.

Roger's exercise consists of walking several times per week. He doesn't do any weight training, but works in the yard and does some household maintenance.

Roger is heavily involved in local marketing associations. He is also a member of several non- profit groups and president of one of these. Roger is heavily involved in local chapters of the American Marketing Association and the society for marketing professional services. In addition he is involved with two local Chambers of Commerce.

At age 67 Roger had been happily married for 39 years. He and his wife have lived a fulfilling life, which has included the caregiving to their 35 year old son.

Roger has a $20,000 savings account. His annuity also allows him to take out emergency withdrawals. Roger chose the annuity for simplicity, security of a guaranteed amount, and it had an acceptable death benefit. If he outlives the principle amount the annuity keeps paying Roger until he dies. If Roger passes on before the principle amount is used, this amount would go to his heirs.

History leading to Retirement

Roger was born in Monterey, California in 1949. Roger travelled to several army bases with his family because his Dad was in the Army. By fourth grade Roger's family finally settled in central Illinois. Roger was the second of four children. There were 2 brothers and a younger sister. The youngest member of the family, a brother, died of colon cancer in his late 40's.

All through school Roger considered himself to be a "nerd". He was in the chess club, science club, and graduated from high school in the top 10%. He did not participate in sports and did very little dating other than a few high school dances. He excelled in math and science.

Although Roger was introverted, he did mingle well with all groups of students while in high school. One of his high school friends influenced Roger into going into engineering in college. This friend would have also gone into engineering, but he soon learned while taking high school calculus that he did not have the aptitude for engineering.

After successfully graduating from High School, Roger went to college locally to obtain his freshman year courses. At the encouraging of his high school counselor, Roger then enrolled in North Western University. He entered a 4 year co-op program.

Roger majored in electrical engineering and did a co-op program for 4 years with General Telephone in Wilmington, Illinois.   Roger was the first co-op student that was hired by General Telephone.   He stayed with General Telephone for six years.

Roger met Diane in the mid 70's. She worked as a ward clerk and admissions clerk for the local hospital. They married in 1977 and spent several years travelling on vacations. They spent their honeymoon in Europe. They went to Hawaii. Just before they married they purchased a small house together.

The first four years of marriage were good. They enjoyed living and working. Then in 1981 their son was born. Initially everything looked good, but after 4 months their family physician noted an anomaly and recommended a specialist.

The specialist noted a major problem with their son that made him intellectually and physically impaired for the rest of his life. He would live well into old age, but be dependent on someone for the rest of his life. He would be in diapers for the remainder of his life.

Roger and Dianne became excellent caregivers, but their carefree and easy life was over. Their life style would revolve around their son and his constant care. Roger's personality tests indicated a desire to help others and Roger has been doing this all his life in addition to his caring for his son.

After working for General Telephone for six years, Roger changed jobs. He accepted a project manager's position with a start-up company that manufactured telecommunications equipment. They were located in Sarasota, Florida. He remained with them until 1987 when he was laid off.

For the next 11 months Roger remained unemployed. Finally, after piling up many bills a head hunter found him an excellent position with Blount Energy Resource Company in Montgomery, Alabama. This Montgomery group was involved with turnkey projects involving converting trash into energy.

He remained with them for 4 years. The trash to energy business did not do well and Roger was laid off after only 4 years. He had been the marketing manager of the group. The entire group was laid off.

After another period of unemployment, Roger accepted a marketing position with BE&K, an industrial engineering and construction company. Roger remained with BE&K for four years until BE&K went through a major transition. Roger then started his own marketing company.

One of his main clients with his new company was in the industrial controls service industry. They and Roger hit it off from the beginning. After 7 months of being on his own they hired him directly.

Roger remained with this last company for 18 years, far longer than any previous company. During his tenure with this company they went from doing around $10 million per year to over $40 million. This made them one of the largest companies in their industry. Roger was in charge of marketing this entire duration. He developed and handled all their marketing collateral materials. He provided a branding program twice during his tenure. Roger was also in charge of all the trade shows and displays and display materials for this company. He was integral in all new products developed by this industrial company.

When he did retire, they offered him a part time position that he is currently involved with.   Roger remained pragmatic his entire career. He only purchased used cars. He did as many of his home repairs as possible. He lived in a very modest two story home. He and his wife did very little traveling after their son was born. His son had severe allergies that precluded plane traffic. They never again left the country.

Retirement Years (Beyond 67)

Roger is barely 68 and has just retired from full time employment. He is currently working part time (20 hours per month) with his previous employer. He is actively pursuing other clients for content development and marketing work opportunities. So far he has picked up one short term client that paid him $5,000.

Roger is also very involved in non-profit activities and is planning on increasing these activities with his new found spare time. With his new spare time, Roger is beginning to write, he is working on landscaping his home, doing other yard work, creating digital art, exploring digital music, and is contemplating doing some fishing.

Lifelong Monetary Plan

Roger's lifelong monetary plan was to pay off his bills and live as frugally as possible. He depended on his 401k for savings.   When he retired from full time employment he converted his 401k to an annuity that pays him $270 per month. He and his wife's main extravagance was their monthly date night.   They would do something each month, usually just a movie. They also had Holiday meals. His monthly mortgage is only $800 per month.

Plan for the Future

Roger's plans for the future mostly include obtaining part time work.   He plans to establish a client base for writing services through marketing activities. He plans to sponsor local marketing association meetings to get his name out there in the marketplace. Roger plans to establish a personal web site to additionally market himself along with regular posts and activity on LinkedIn.

Roger plans to continue his annual family vacations with his relatives. Each year one relative is in charge of picking a location and organizing the group food and vacation activities. Each member pays his or her own way.

One thing that Roger is not necessarily counting on or preparing for is a likely possibility to receive a large inheritance (approximately $500,000-$1,000,000) from his wife's family. This inheritance is in the form of land worth approximately $2 million dollars. His wife and her brother would equally share this inheritance.

This would change his life from adequate financially to comfortable. They would hire a Nanny to travel with them to take care of their son. Roger and his wife have only briefly talked about what they would do with this inheritance. He has not looked into what this could mean in a monthly income. He has thought he might use part of this money to remodel his house which he estimates would equate to approximately 50,000.

If he does inherit land worth a million dollars, this will likely change his life dramatically. He hasn't really thought about it, but one way or another his life will change with this inheritance.

SWOT Analysis

Strengths:

Roger's greatest strength lies in his large network of business associates and friends. In addition, his health and financial resources are good. Writing skills and marketing knowledge that is saleable to various customer groups is also a major plus.

Weaknesses:

His part time work with his old company could come to an end. His old company is already moving others into doing the work that Roger is currently doing.

Opportunities:

Roger's greatest opportunities lie in his obtaining new clients and a client list for future work. His work with non-profits could also lead to paid for work in this arena. He also as mentioned has the potential for a windfall inheritance of approximately one million dollars. This would be a life changer.

Threats:

As mentioned under the weakness section, his current part time work with his ex-employer could dry up. He could also not find any significant business with new clients.

Civic Activities

Roger has taken several personality tests in the course of his life and career. All of these tests show that Roger has a high propensity for servicing others. This propensity has been channeled into several civic and non-profits that Roger works with.

Regrets

Everyone has some regrets. Roger regrets never having learned to play a musical instrument. He had an opportunity in the 6th grade when his parents asked him if he was interested. Roger declined and regrets this loss of opportunity.

Chapter 4
(Mary)

Name	Age	Education	Financial Strength	Health	Age Last Worked	Plan Strength
Mary	94	High Sch.	Moderate	Failed	65	N.A.

Overview

Mary recently passed away. Mary outlived two husbands. She had two sons by her first marriage and none by her second. The elder son, who had moved out at age 18 had 5 children and lived in Pensacola, Florida. Her youngest son lived near Mary. He had lived with his mother into his late 20's. He was gay and eventually started living with a gay lover.

Her first husband died young of a massive heart attack at age 49. Mary was also 49. Within 3 years she married her second husband, who then passed away at 74 when Mary was 62.

Mary worked for the three years between husbands. Her first husband had left her fairly well off. She wasn't rich, but she was able to continue her life style in Pelham, New York. Mary helped her second son with a book that he was writing for High School English.

Mary was a legal secretary. Her fingers had the onset of arthritis and it had become difficult for Mary to keep up with the typing requirements at age 62. Even so, she managed and still was an excellent worker and well thought of by the law firm.

After Phil passed away Mary lived by herself until she was 89 and then moved in with her younger son. He obtained power of attorney and took all of Mary's assets including a fund that Mary had set out for her eldest son with his name on the account along with Mary's.

The elder son was to receive these funds ($75,000) at the death of Mary and the youngest son was to obtain the family house. But the youngest son, Ralph, emptied the account with his power of attorney. Mary had warned the older son that the younger was after the money. There was nothing the older son could do. And he was not about to hire a lawyer to sue a relative.

The youngest son then sold the family house for $800,000 cash. Mary is probably turning over in her grave at this injustice. She died of Alzheimer's disease the same month as her 94th birthday.

Mary's second husband lived in Mary's house and paid the bills. He left a significant stock portfolio for Mary. The dividends from these stocks and bonds were to go to Mary for the balance of her life. Upon Mary's death these stocks and bonds were to be transferred to Phil's three children from his first marriage.

Although Phil had left these dividends for Mary, Mary had difficulty in her late 80's meeting her house taxes. Her younger son stepped in to help, but insisted that half of the house be turned over to him with the rest to go to him at Mary's death. At this time he also convinced Mary to give him power of attorney.

Situation at Age 67

At age 67, Mary's second husband had been dead for 5 years. As mentioned, Mary received the dividends from Phil's stocks and bonds. This coupled with social security and some saved money left Mary able to pay her bills and live modestly until she was in her middle 80's when inflation and rising house taxes caught up with her. But at 67 she was doing okay.

Mary enjoyed a fairly rich social life. She remained close to Phil's three children and enjoyed seeing them at their homes. She also had them over to her house. She also had her younger son, who lived nearby. They ate together at least once per week.

She also belonged to a club that met every Tuesday. She would get involved in some of the activities of the club. Each Tuesday they had a luncheon at their fine clubhouse. They participated in social and civic activities.

Financially, at age 67, Mary had the following income:

Social S. --	$15,200
Dividends--	$11,000
Interest --	$ 4,500
Boarder--	$ 6,000
Total	$36,700

The interest came from her inheritance from her father. He left her the house, which netted her $75,000 when it was sold. In the 1970's and 1980's this annual income was sufficient to meet Mary's needs. At the age of 67, she had no mortgage on the house and her taxes had not gone up to the extent that they would later on. Mary had no real expenses other than food and clothes and gifts for relatives at birthdays and Christmas.

Physically Mary was in good shape. She had had eye surgery for cataracts and could actually see 20-20. She did smoke, but only a few cigarettes a day. She had been smoking since she was 33. She drank a glass of wine each day. She rarely had colds and did not have blood pressure or cholesterol issues.

She would spend part of her late spring at her elder son's water front cottages in Gulf Shores, Alabama. Her elder son had two cottages that were next to each other. Mary would bring a friend and her family. The friend and family would stay in the other cottage. They did this for many years.

History leading to Retirement

Mary was born in Yonkers, New York in 1920. Her parents were from Italy. Her father was a plasterer and maintenance worker. She grew up with two younger brothers. Her mother worked in the home and raised the children. They were relatively poor.

Mary was a good student in school. She studied to be a secretary and did very well. When she was 20 she was working in Manhattan in a secretarial pool. She lived at home to help support her parents. Her father was unable to obtain full time employment for a while during this time.

Mary was an excellent worker with a strong work ethic. She would come into work no matter what the conditions. One time when the snow in Yonkers was up to her knees in places, she walked to the train station early in the morning to make work.

She started taking night classes at John's Hopkins University, but she was only able to take a few courses to help her secretarial work. But at this night school she met her future husband. They married when Mary was 22. Her husband dropped out of school and became a successful salesman. They enjoyed their first 5 years without children. Their first child was born when Mary was 30.

From the age of 22 to 30 Mary and her husband enjoyed the life in Manhattan. They lived there and enjoyed the night club life. They took vacations and went to dude ranches and other vacation spots.

They weren't rich by any stretch of the imagination, but they lived modestly in a one bedroom apartment. They had friends that they played cards with every week. They did things as a foursome and sometimes six or even eight got together, especially for cards during the week.

Mary had a second child when she was 36. Their one bedroom apartment became too small for four people so they built a two bedroom home in Pelham, New York. She was 38 when they moved to Pelham.

Mary had never driven a car before. Living in New York one did not need a car because of the public transportation. She lived within short walking distance of subway, trolley cars, trains, and buses. She could get on the bus and be at her parent's house in the suburbs in under an hour.

She could and did walk to the stores that were on the same block as the apartment that they lived in. Within 4 blocks there was a butcher store, grocery, hardware, jewelry store, movie theater, and several dress shops. Everything necessary for Mary's growing family.

However, at the age of 38, living in Pelham required being able to drive a car. She could not drive a "shift car" so her husband purchased an automatic drive car for her. So at the ripe age of 38 she went to driving school. She obtained her license and drove until she was 87. She never had an accident in all her years of driving.

Mary became a civic minded person. She worked at the grade school that her younger child attended. She volunteered there and at numerous other civic organizations. She eventually joined the "Manor Club", which was a social and civics club that had its own clubhouse. The women of the town met there every Tuesday for a lunch meeting. This group was involved with many philanthropic activities.

Mary's two sons were diametrically opposite in nature. The older son was extremely independent. He would join Little League and just in passing mention it to his parents. He managed to get to the games on his own. He was gone from home until dinnertime each day. He preferred to be out with friends, playing baseball or whatever was in season.

On the other hand the younger son was almost anti-social. He preferred to remain at home growing up. Mary spent a great deal of time with him. She hired a psychologist to evaluate the younger son because he was so anti-social. Mary hovered over him and ignored the older son. The older son was happy to be left to his own devices. He was wild, but managed to keep one step ahead of getting into serious trouble.

Both sons did well in school, although the younger son was much more scholastic and conscientious. They both went to college and they both graduated. The older son just made it with barely passing grades in 4 years of college and then went directly to marriage and work.

The older son worked from early age. He worked through college to defray the expense of school. The younger son did not work until after he went to graduate school. He became a teacher, but this did not last long. For some reason he left his teaching position.

Mary worked with him to develop with two other writers, English grammar books for high school students. The three writers did very well.

It is not clear when Mary learned that her younger son was Gay. She tried to hide the fact for most of her life. She invented girl boy relations for the younger son. She would intimate that he did not marry because it was later in life that he had been able to afford a wife. She never told the older son, but eventually he figured it out.

The older son was living a thousand miles away and only had occasional yearly contact with Mary and his younger brother. In addition, he was busy with his career and marriage and three sons for most of this time. When he did meet with Mary and his younger brother, Mary made sure that her younger son had a date that she could parade in front of the older brother.

It was always the same girl. She was a "friend only" of the younger brother. In fact after she married, Mary still referred to this girl and her younger son as a couple. The older son, not being around much did not catch onto the lack of a true male-female love interest. Mary kept her younger son's secret life very well.

At the time of her first husband's death Mary's older son was three months from college graduation. Right after graduation he married and moved several states away. Mary had enough money from life insurance, social security, and the sale of her husband's air conditioning business and assets to remain in her life style.

As mentioned, she remarried 3 years later to a man 12 years her senior. The greatest thing that this marriage provided was additional security for Mary. Her new husband, Phil, moved into Mary's home and paid the bills.

In addition to security this second marriage provided a social life. Phil had three children living in the area. Each was married with several children of their own. Since this was a close family, they were always getting together. Mary truly enjoyed these get togethers.

In addition, her new husband liked to travel. He was retired. He had sold his business. He had been a sub-contractor involved with demolition of buildings. He played golf. Mary learned to play golf and enjoyed their trips. During their marriage, one of Phil's daughters moved to Arizona. So they enjoyed going out west to visit her and her family as well.

They travelled to Tennessee to visit Mary's oldest son. He moved to North Carolina and they visited him there as well. They had a busy retirement and enjoyed their relatives and friends. And they enjoyed their travels.

Then at age 76 Phil developed leukemia. Mary was only 63 when he died. She took care of Phil right up to the end. Mary went back to work as a legal secretary until she reached 65 and then retired.

Retirement Years (67 and beyond)

Mary lived alone for the next 22 years (67-89) until she developed Dementia and then Alzheimer's. During this 22 year period, she continued to enjoy her second husband's children and their children even though he was now deceased. This extended family was a major part of Mary's life. She continued her Tuesday sessions with the Manor Club and met her younger son for dinner several times a month.

Mary's second husband had converted the family den and put a room in the attic with a shower. The den had a half bath and this two room part of the house made an excellent living quarters for a boarder. Mary took in a lovely woman who liked living alone. For the remainder of her life, Mary had the income from this boarder.

Mary also visited with her eldest son and his children also visited Mary during this time. Although Mary lived alone she had an active social life. However, during this time all of Mary's friends and peers of the same age had died.

As discussed, Mary managed financially until her middle 80's when her younger son had to step in and help with the taxes. For this he obtained the house and all of Mary's assets. Then at 89 she moved in with her youngest son. He hired caregivers to help Mary for the last two years of her life. He kept her in a "bonus room" upstairs that was only approximately 6 ft. by 7 ft. He rarely went up to see her.

When she died, she only had a small group of family and friends attend the funeral. The elder son said a few words over the grave, but no one else was able to say anything at the grave site. The eldest son told of a time that he remembered an incident that reflected Mary's strength of character. Both the younger son and Mary's youngest brother tried, but couldn't say any words. It was a drizzly cold winter's day at the gravesite when Mary was laid to rest.

SWOT Analysis

Strengths:

Since Mary is now deceased, I cannot talk about her future in a SWOT analysis. I will go back in time to her retirement years starting at age 67 and progressing to 94 and perform the analysis from this vantage point. Mary's strength comes from having a paid up house and an income from her second husband's estate. She also had the income from a boarder who remained at the home for the duration of Mary's life.

She is also fortunate to have two sons who are financially sound. One son will eventually help with the house taxes and will take her into his house at the end of her life. The other son provided Mary with paid vacations to Gulf Shores, Alabama.

Also, her second husband's family provided Mary with a strong social outlet. Mary was also fortunate to be able to stay in her home. She had the Manor Club within walking distance as an additional social outlet.

Weaknesses:

Mary lived alone for her retirement years. With no one in the house to help her, she was in the position of having a major accident with no one to help her.   In her late 80's she developed Alzheimer's disease.

Opportunities:

Mary had enough money, family, friends, and social life to live comfortably into her mid 80's.   She had the opportunity for a rich social life between family, friends, and the Manor Club. She took full advantage of these.

Threats:

Looking back, Mary had a relatively healthy life until she developed Alzheimer's disease.   This was her main threat. Inflation was her second threat and it caught up with her in her late 80's in the form of property taxes.   Also, her home was getting old and needed a new roof.

Civic Activities

The majority of Mary's civic activities revolved around the activities that she involved herself in with the Manor Club in Pelham.

Regrets

Mary's greatest regret is that her first husband died so young. He was only 49 when he died of a massive heart attack. She also regretted that neither of her sons became doctors or lawyers, although they were both very successful in their fields.

Mary also regretted that her youngest son was gay. She tried to hide this fact from the world for the majority of her life. It bothered her immensely.

Mary may have had other regrets, but these were her most critical regrets.

Chapter 5
(Clete)

Name	Age	Education	Financial Strength	Health	Age Last Worked	Plan Strength
Clete	98	High Sch.	Moderate	Rough	69 yrs	N.A.

Overview

Clete was born in 1919 and as of the writing of this book is still alive. He is living in a nursing home 50 miles north of New York City. The cost for this nursing home is $12,750 per month. The cost has become prohibitive and so Clete is being taken in by his eldest daughter. They will all live in Clete's old home. It is a small two bedroom home in a lovely section of Buchanan, New York.

Clete has been an independent person all his life. The idea of college never entered his mind. He went straight to work after he left the eighth grade. He felt that he had learned all he needed by the eighth grade.

One of the things that made Clete unique in life was his spending each winter in Florida (Fort Myers). After he sold his juke box and pin ball business , he purchased a trailer and each winter he and his wife would travel from Buchanan, New York to Florida and take up residency until spring.

Clete met his wife while working as a teenager in a bakery near his home. His wife was the daughter of the owners of the bakery.

Clete's boyhood home was within walking distance of the Yonkers, New York Racetrack. This racetrack was Westchester County's horse racing and betting mecca. Today it also sports a gambling casino.

At the bakery, Clete met his first wife. His first wife was his soul mate. While Clete was not faithful to his wife, he had a respect for her and maintained a semblance of marriage until she died in her mid-70's.

Clete's work life was interesting. While he worked for others in his early career, he soon branched off into many small business endeavors. One of which was a juke box and pinball machine business.

In the juke box and pin ball business, Clete utilized his younger brother and his brother in law as employees. His business did extremely well. When he sold it, he was virtually able to coast through many more ventures with a nice financial cushion. When his eldest daughter had to step in with power of attorney to handle his estate in Clete's late 90's, she learned that Clete had accumulated in several banks almost $750,000 dollars. Clete was a self-made man.

Clete always lived frugally. He bought a small home in Dobbs Ferry, New York shortly after he married his first wife. Sometime after his daughter was born in 1943 they moved to Buchanan, New York where Clete purchased a slightly larger home.

In his neighborhood, Clete was not well liked. However, in his work with Airstream Trailers and his trips to Florida with his Airstream, he became involved with the Airstream Club. The club members all owned Airstream trailers and traveled as a group to different places. He was popular with them.

Clete and his wife would go with them to many locations throughout the U.S. If the club called him up and he was in the middle of a project, he would put it on hold and hit the road with the group. Sometimes for as long as 3 months at time they would travel the roads.

Situation at Age 67

Right after Clete turned 67 he and his wife were on an airstream trip. Their youngest daughter, Cloe, had just graduated from high school. Clete and his wife thought she would do like the older daughter and get married and move off.

However, Clete and his wife received a call that their daughter planned on jumping to her death from a nearby cliff. They hurried home to talk with her. Clete's wife wanted to hire a psychiatrist, but Clete didn't believe in psychiatry.

They did hire one for a while. He interviewed the family members and said that Clete was a sadist. This was strange and Clete put his foot down and said he would handle his youngest daughter. He immediately bought a Pontiac convertible and a small motorcycle for her. He also agreed to pay fully for her to go to college.

So Cloe went off to college in Sarasota. She didn't do very well. In fact she dropped out after a year. But the delay had worked and Cloe no longer threatened suicide. She did indeed then get married and has had a reasonably good life.

At age 67 (age of retirement) Clete was doing well. He had accumulated a good deal of money (approximately $300,000) and had a fair income. Clete's wife also had a business selling jewelry that she made from materials purchased in the lower west side of Manhattan and brought back to Westchester. She had a route that she had developed where she sold this jewelry to stores on her route.

Clete at this time was a real estate agent and he also purchased old homes, fixed them up, and sold them. He was doing quite well. Financially, at age 67, Clete had the following income:

Social S. --	$6,706	(Clete)
Social S.	$3,353	(Wife)
Real Estate	$6,000	
Home Turnover	$4,500	
Jewelry Bus.	$3,500	
Interest Income	$30,000	
Miscellaneous	$3,000	
Total	$57,059	

Clete had virtually no real outgo other than his trips and food. He had paid off his mortgage. His two girl children were grown. He had no debts. He owned a very inexpensive home in Buchanan and a permanent trailer in a trailer park in Fort Myers.

Interest rates on jumbo cd's were still 10% in 1986 when Clete was 67. However, they plummeted over the next couple of years down to current rates just over 1%. Clete's interest income would fall dramatically, but he would still continue to add to his savings each year at the average of $14,000 per year.

His miscellaneous income came from Clete's ability to always turn a dollar. When copper prices sky rocketed, he would go to factory "bone yards" and scrap piles and buy the waste copper products cheap. He would then sell the copper portion of these pieces on the open market place.

Socially, Clete and his wife still wintered in Florida where they had developed friendships. They also continued to take Airstream trips with the Airstream Club.

At 67 they had friends, they had security, and they had a life. Added to this, Clete had a mistress that he kept quiet. She was the wife of a local Buchanan dentist. This affair had been going on for many years. Other than the problem with their youngest daughter that Clete had handled his way, things were good for Clete.

History Leading to Retirement

Clete grew up in Yonkers, New York. He was the middle sibling. He had a sister 6 years older and a brother 6 years younger. His father was a construction worker who drifted into plastering. His mother was a housewife. When he was growing up they lived in a garage for a while. During this time Clete's father built a modest house that they finally moved into.

When Clete was seven years old he was an altar boy in a Catholic Church. One day Clete was climbing a tree to pick an apple. This tree was on church property. The priest saw Clete and called him down from the tree. This priest then dismissed Clete from being an altar boy.

Whatever possessed this priest to inflict such a harsh punishment for such an innocent activity is beyond belief. Unfortunately it had a major impact on Clete. He never went back inside a church and he lost respect for authority figures. Clete did well in his business endeavors, but he disliked and did not respect anyone of authority.

Clete and his family lived near the Yonkers Race Track. When Clete was barely a teenager he would sneak out at night and go to the race track.

Early in the depression years Clete's family lost the house because they could not keep up the payments. However, they did get some money from the sale of this house. It was enough for Clete's father to build another house later in Ardsley, New York. But by this time Clete was gone.

Clete's last schooling was the 8th grade. He dropped out of school because he felt that further education was wasted. During his teen years Clete had many different jobs. The one that had its greatest impact was a job working in a bakery in nearby Tuckahoe. At this point Clete was 18 years of age and working in this bakery. The owners of the bakery had a very pretty daughter one year younger than Clete.

In 1939 at the age of 20 Clete married Dorothy. She was the daughter of the bakery owners. Clete moved in with Dorothy in her parent's home. They were living there during the 1940 census. Since Dorothy's parents owned a bakery Clete and

Dorothy worked in the bakery. They didn't make much money, but they had a roof over their heads and a place to work.

Clete bought a small home in Dobbs Ferry, New York shortly after the 1940 census. Sometime after his daughter was born in 1943 they moved to Buchanan, New York where Clete purchased a slightly larger home.

Clete's parents came from Italy and Dorothy's parents were German. In 1940 this was an unusual combination. In 1943 Pete and Dorothy had their first of two girl children. They named her after her mother. Baby Dorothy helped keep Clete from becoming involved with World War II. He was already exempt because after the bakery sold he went to work for a company involved in the war effort.

During the war years Clete worked shift work at North American Phillips in Briarcliff Manor, New York. North American Phillips manufactured gyroscopes for gun sights on fighter planes. At the time men who worked in defense related industries were deferred from the draft. Clete's mother was upset that her younger son was drafted and Clete was not.

Clete never had a good relationship with his parents. It was rumored that Pete was not his father's real son. Clete's mother ran off for a period. When she returned she was pregnant with another man's child. This other man died in an influenza epidemic (flu pandemic of 1918 which destroyed 1/3 of the world's population) in late 1918 or early 1919. Clete was born in 1919.

The details were sketchy, but Clete's mother said that Clete had a "black heart". Many years later when Clete's father (one who raised him) died he disinherited Clete. He had willed his home, which sold for $100,000 to his daughter and Clete's younger brother. The daughter netted $75,000 and the younger son received $25,000 per the will's percentages. The daughter obtained the larger percentage because she had helped the family financially many times over the years.

At the end of WWII, Clete no longer was able to work for North American Philips. He then went into several endeavors. He started an upholstery shop where he did fine work. At some point he got into the repairing and supplying of juke boxes and pin ball machines.

He expanded this into supplying these units to bars and restaurants on a "split the revenue" basis. He hired his younger brother and also utilized his brother in law to collect the money in the juke boxes and pin ball machines. The younger brother also delivered the units to these establishments.

His younger brother was an electronics technician. He had learned electronics in the navy. In the navy he had been schooled in electronics and was the ships radio man (Broadcast Operator). When he got out of the navy he held odd jobs for several years before going to work for Clete. He also became a ham radio operator. He built his own radio station.

Clete used him to fix the pin ball and juke boxes as well as collect the money in the boxes as previously mentioned. These boxes were installed on a "split the revenue" basis with their various customers. The collected revenue would be split and ratioed with the owners of the establishments.

One potential customer that had more machines than anyone else was a gaming installation on Central Avenue in Yonkers. They had 50 or more units. Young teenagers and even older people would go into this establishment and spend hours on the pin ball machines. They would put their quarters in the machines. Clete wanted to get this customer for his own business. So one day he and his younger brother Billy went in there to meet the owner manager.

The owner manager told Clete and Billy that he wasn't interested in making a change. Clete wouldn't be put off. He asked if any of the units were broken. He told the owner that Billy was a genius at repair and would be glad to look at any unit that wasn't working.

It so happened that there was a bad unit. This unit could be adding revenue if it could be fixed. So the owner let Billy look at it. Billy took it apart and was trying to figure out what was wrong with it.

It was Clete however that noticed a wire that was "loose". It wasn't disconnected, just loose from its solder joint. Clete had Billy go to his car and get a soldering gun and some solder. This turned out to be the problem and fixed the pin ball machine. The owner wanted to pay Clete, but Clete refused. He just said that next time he had a need to please call Clete's company. This opened up a new customer over time, a very large one.

Clete's success in the juke box and pin ball business didn't go unnoticed. A group of well healed gangsters from New York wanted to "horn in" on the action. They used intimidation tactics to get Clete to sell all or part of his business to them. They would show up in Clete's driveway and intimidate his family.

Clete contacted the FBI. The FBI gave Clete and his family a number to call whenever these gangsters would appear. It became a cat and mouse game with the gangsters continuing to intimidate Clete. He just wouldn't be intimidated. His family was scared, but Clete continued to operate his business as usual.

Finally, these gangsters from New York offered Clete a sweet financial deal to sell his company. Clete negotiated with them and sold his business for a good deal of money—over $200,000 cash. This was more money than Clete had ever seen.

In the 1960's this was a great deal of money. It then gave Clete capital to start other businesses. One of these was the nursery business. Clete gave his brother in law Tad a part of his money from the sale of the juke box business. He did this in order to become a partner in Tad's nursery start-up business.

Tad had gone to a two year college in horticulture. He developed and learned a great deal with which to start the nursery business. He also had some capital from the sale of his mother's bakery. When Clete approached Tad about going in together in the nursery business, Tad turned Clete down. He felt that Clete had nothing to offer.

So Clete decided to open his own nursery business. Clete was very smart, but not smart enough. He used land around his home to develop the plants and flowers for his nursery. Clete's nursery was only marginally successful. Clete soon abandoned this business.

Retirement Years (Beyond 67)

Clete had sold his juke box business and this money ($200,000) served him well. He would loan out money at good rates (for him). He had abandoned his nursery business. He started making small trailers to attach to cars. This business was marginally successful, so he broadened it to repairing and selling Airstream trailers.

From the Airstream business, Clete developed a relationship with the Airstream Club. He and his wife would travel all over the U.S. in caravan style with the Airstream Club.

Clete purchased a bar and restaurant that he and his wife ran for a while. They then turned it over to his oldest daughter and her husband.

Clete then became a real estate agent. While he was an agent he would be keenly aware of "fixer uppers". Clete would purchase these, fix them up, and sell them at a profit. One of these units was directly behind his home.

It was on a quiet cull de sac. Clete and his wife lived in their trailer on the new property while he was fixing it up. He had sold his original home for a nice profit. He was in the middle of refurbishing the house when the Airstream club called about a month long motor trip. Clete and his wife put the refurbishment on hold and took off with the club.

Clete and his wife still wintered in Fort Myers, Florida. And they still travelled with the Airstream Club. But at the age of 75, Clete's wife died. She had developed a terminal cancer. Clete now 76 was devastated. Even though Clete had been unfaithful, he had also been discreet and loved his first wife. He stayed with her in the hospital night and day until she died.

During their years of wintering in Florida and travelling with the Airstream club Clete and his wife had become good friends with another travelling husband and wife who lived in New Jersey. It so happened that the wife (Barbara) of this couple had recently lost her husband. So Clete and she got together and eventually married.

Clete continued to do odd jobs including grounds keeper in the trailer park in Fort Myers. Eventually his second wife wanted to live on the family property in New Jersey. By this time they were both in their 90's. He abandoned his home in Buchanan and moved to New Jersey.

The second wife's family had a small building on the property that was fixed up and used as Clete's and his wife's residence. This residence was close to the main house in which the rest of the family lived.

In the meantime, Clete's oldest daughter with her significant other moved into Clete's abandoned house. It was going to ruin and they had much to do to get it back to a working home. Clete continued to live in New Jersey with Barbara on her family's property.

When Clete was in his late 90's Barbara had a major stroke and had to be placed in a nursing home. Shortly afterwards, Clete's older daughter received a call from one of the family members in the main house. It was late on a snowy evening. The family member informed the daughter that she was to come and get her father immediately. The family could not be responsible for Clete's safety.

Apparently, Clete did not like living in New Jersey. He would defecate and urinate on the property. This was not out of age, but out of meanness. At least that is what the oldest daughter determined. At any rate, the oldest daughter travelled the 3 hour trip in the snow early the next morning and picked up her father.

Clete stayed with his oldest daughter for six months. After six months they had to put him in a nursing home. The first home they put him in was not very good and so they moved him to a better and more expensive home.

He is still in this home, but the monthly cost ($12,750) is becoming a drain on Clete's resources. So the plan is to move him back into his old home and his daughter who is an RN will take care of him. As she puts it, "he can camp out in the living room."

So at over 98 years of age, Clete will be coming home and his daughter will look after him. If Clete lives to be 100 he will be the first and only one to reach this age in his family.

Lifelong Monetary Plan

Clete had a lifelong monetary plan. It was work from early age (8th grade) and turn a profit on any endeavor that he could think of. Clete was in retail baking, worked in a defense plant during the war, had a juke box and pin ball machine company, nursery business, real estate, refurbished homes, built trailers, provided Airstream repair and sales, copper and aluminum sales, and upholstery business to name a few of his endeavors.

He lived frugally, yet still had a life. He wintered in Florida in a motor home that was then upgraded to a permanent trailer on a trailer lot he purchased. He didn't fool with stocks or bonds. He mostly used banks and jumbo CD's. During the 70's and early 80's he capitalized on high interest rates.

As of right now, Clete still has a nice savings that his oldest daughter is handling with power of attorney.

Plan for the Future

Clete's plan for the future is day to day to stay alive. He no longer can work or turn a dollar. He will come home and as his daughter says "camp out in the living room". When he does pass this life his grave stone should read from the Frank Sinatra song "I did it my way".

SWOT Analysis

Strengths:

Clete's strength lies in his large bank balance, lack of debts, and a daughter who is an RN and willing to take him into her home (Clete's old home). In his life, Clete's initial strength came from his wife's family's retail bakery and his ability to turn a profit in his endeavors.

His strength then came from getting into the juke box and pin ball business at just the right time and then selling it at just the right time for a handsome profit. Clete had a high energy and a knack for turning a profit in virtually every endeavor.

Weaknesses:

Obviously, at this point Clete's main weakness is his age and health. It is very difficult for someone who has been extremely active all his life to see his body deteriorating.

Opportunities:

The opportunity that Clete has is to live out the rest of his life in relative comfort with his daughter in his old home.

Threats:

Sharing a small house with a relative can be trying at any age. At an elderly age it can be even more trying.

Civic Activities

It is not likely that Clete participated in any civic activities.

Regrets

Clete lived his life on his own terms. His only regret that we know of is that he is no longer physically strong enough to do the things that he would like to do.

Health Issues

At almost 99, health is the issue. Clete had a relatively healthy and long life, but he is weak now and not able to do the things he would like to. He has diabetes, high blood pressure, COPD and other ailments that he takes pills for. He can no longer walk. He is weak and mostly sits or sleeps.

Chapter 6
(Angie)

Name	Age	Education	Financial Strength	Health	Age Last Worked	Plan Strength
Angie	79	High Schl.	Weak	Fair	60 yrs	Fair

Overview

Angie is a 79 year old widow. She was born in Chicago and spent her early grade school years growing up close to the Cubs stadium. In fact she could walk to the stadium from her house.

Her family moved several times to find work. Angie's family wasn't dirt poor, but her family just got by. However, Angie didn't lack for anything. She always had a roof over her head and food to eat. She received toys at Christmas.

After several moves to find work they settled in Sunnyland Illinois where Angie graduated from high school. In high school she met and fell in love with her soon to be husband, William. They married and had a child right out of high school.

They rented homes the first 2 1/2 years of their marriage and then purchased a townhouse. This townhouse was the middle house of three connected units. They raised their 3 children there. They paid the unit off in 1961.

William worked for a tool and die company called H.M. Harper's for many years until they closed up. He worked their during the week and worked at a gas station on the week-ends. When Harper's closed, he then went to work for a small company in Skokie, which is about 15 miles from Chicago.

Angie worked for an insurance company called Benefit Trust Insurance Company. She worked with them for over 10 years. She worked there long enough to obtain a small pension.

After over 30 years of marriage they finally bought their own home in Trevor, Wisconsin about 50 miles from Skokie. It was an older prefab house that was on a large lot. At this time, William was working for a new company and was well liked by this company.

However, shortly after going to work for this new company and shortly after purchasing their home, William developed a terminal cancer. He died two years later in 1995.

Angie had to rent part of her home to make ends meet. She had this income for many years into her retirement. However, her boarder died two years ago. Her retirement years will be covered in the section titled "Retirement Years (Beyond 67). Angie had to rely on a reverse mortgage that she obtained two years ago. The details of the reverse mortgage will also be covered in the "Retirement Years" section.

Angie at 79 has all her faculties, although she has some issues that slow her down some. She no longer has a car and must rely on family, friends, and wheels for seniors to get around.

She lives alone and handles her affairs. Next month she will have cataract surgery. She is very brave about it. She knows she needs the surgery because her doctor has said she does. She also cannot read without employing a Sherlock Holmes type magnifying glass.

At age 79, Angie just gets by with her income and outgo. She lives extremely frugally and with her reverse mortgage is coping with the unexpected bills so far.

Situation at Age 67

In the year 2004, Angie was 67 years of age. Her husband had been dead for 9 years. She had a renter (boarder) who lived in her house and contributed to expenses. He did not pay a monthly amount, but contributed food and food stamps, paid the utilities, and provided whatever support he could. If his payments were paid in a monthly rental they would equal approximately $400 per month.

At age 67 Angie was in her own home. She paid a monthly mortgage of $707.72 and received help with expenses from her boarder. By receiving help with expenses Angie did not have to count this as rental income on her income tax.

Financially, Angie had 4 incomes each year as follows:

Social S. --	$14,772
Angie pension	$ 1,968
Husband's pension	$ 1,632
Renter's contribution	$ 4,800
Total	$ 23.172

Angie's main outgo was her mortgage at $9,248.64 per year. This left her only $13,923 to live on for the year. This amounted to $1,160 per month. However, out of this comes $340/month for taxes and insurance. In the year 2004 this was almost enough to live on comfortably. She was managing.

Her renter's contribution is an estimate because as mentioned he helped with bills, but did not pay a monthly fee.

Angie's social life revolved around her children and grandchildren and friends. Two of her children both lived close by. Neither was well off, but they also got by financially.

Angie's health at this time was fair. She had some arthritis in her back, but had not yet developed or noticed that she had the beginnings of COPD. She also had a mild case of high blood pressure.

Angie's pension came from her over 10 years working for Benefit Trust Insurance Company. Her husband's pension came from his last job. These were the days when companies offered pensions to their employees.

Angie's main asset was her home. She had a nice piece of land with a Quonset hut for storage. She also had a fenced space for her three dogs that served her well. Her house had originally been a prize that someone won in a lottery. It was prefabricated. Both the boiler furnace and the hot water heater are extremely old. They are still working, but will eventually require replacement.

Angie still drove and had an older, but reliable car that she drove to the store and to visit friends and relatives. She and her husband mostly purchased used cars. Their car purchases over the years had been in the $1,800 to $3,300 range. However, they did purchase a brand new Pontiac when their children were young. They used this to haul a small 18' trailer that they used for vacations with the kids.

History Leading to Retirement

As mentioned earlier Angie was born and spent her early grade school years growing up in Chicago close to the Cubs stadium.

Her family moved several times to find work. She always had a roof over her head and food to eat. Angie was an only child. Angie was above average in school. As a matter of fact her school wanted to move her ahead a grade or two. However her parents declined because they felt she was socially not ready. She did over time develop a sense of humor and an easy going personality.

Angie left Chicago at the end of the third grade. Her father found work in Cleveland for 6 months and then moved the family to Detroit for a better job. They lived in Detroit for four years. Then her mother's brother knew of a job in Sunnyland, Illinois. So the family packed up and moved for another job.

Angie remembers Sunnyland as a wonderful place with grass and trees. They lived on a dirt road. Most of the roads in Sunnyland were dirt at this time.

She got pregnant and married right as she was graduating from high school. Her husband William was a good supporter, but did not make much money. They rented initially and then purchased a townhouse on the outskirts of Chicago.

While her husband worked for a company that manufactured nuts and bolts, Angie worked for an insurance company. She had two children, a boy and a girl. The boy, Jay, had a friend in the eighth grade whose parents were from Romania.

Her son's friends name was Fen. When Jay and Fen were in the eighth grade Fen's father was shot and killed as he was entering his home. He was shot from the roof of a home across the street. Fen's mother was weak from an illness that had started when she had been held in a concentration camp in Romania.

The murderer of Fen's father was never brought to justice. It was thought that the murderer had shot Fen's father over a Romanian gambling game. It is believed that the murderer moved back to Romania. There was never a resolution to this case.

Fen's mother wasn't strong enough to take care of Fen. The mother died within a year of her husband. So Angie and her husband took Fen in and raised him as their son. He became a successful football player in high school. He then went to a military college for a while and then graduated from Southern Illinois University in Carbondale, Ill.

Fen still refers to Angie as his mother. They keep in touch. Angie is also still close to her other son and daughter. The son lives 18 miles from Angie and the daughter is one hour away. Fen lives in Virginia where he is a liaison for the Army.

William worked for a company that made all sorts of fasteners (nut, bolts, etc.) called H.M. Harper for many years until they closed up. When Harper closed, William lost his future pension. He then went to work for a small company in Skokie on the outskirts of Chicago. When he died this company paid Angie $5,000 and she obtained William's IRA pension of $136.00 per month.

Angie worked for Benefit Trust Insurance Company for over 10 years. This was long enough to obtain a small pension of $164.34 per month.

After many years of marriage they finally bought their own real home in Trevor, Wisconsin about 50 miles from Skokie. It was an older prefab house that was on a large lot.

This house had originally come into being as a prize that was won at the Wisconsin State Fair. It was a prefab called the Wausau. The winner of the prefab house had it delivered and put together in Trevor, Wisconsin in 1964. William and Angie eventually purchased it from him in 1993.

At this time, William was working for a new company and was well liked by this company. However, shortly after going to work for this new company and shortly after purchasing their home, William developed a terminal cancer. He died two years later in 1995.

Angie had to rent part of her home to make ends meet. She had this income for many years into her retirement. However, her boarder died two years ago. Angie then had to rely on a reverse mortgage that she obtained two years ago. The details of the reverse mortgage will be covered in the next section.

Retirement Years (Beyond 67)

Angie was 67 in 2004. Her husband was dead and she was living on social security, two small pensions, and shared expenses with her boarder.

Her boarder died at the beginning of 2015. Angie then started looking at a reverse mortgage as a way to overcome the loss of her boarder's share of living expenses.

Angie's reverse mortgage pays her monthly mortgage of $707.72. So Angie no longer has a mortgage payment. It also provides a pool of money that Angie can draw from. This pool if not used will grow with the interest rate existing at the time. She basically has a net line of credit of $29,366, which grows each month. The previous month was $29,258. This amounts to 3.7% interest, which is much better than a savings account.

She obtained this reverse mortgage with Sunset West in California. She did not go with AIG because she did not like one of the actors that was advertising this product. She felt that he never finished anything he started. He worked in TV and even ran for president for a short time, but he quit on both. Angie had her local credit union help her in putting this reverse mortgage together.

The reverse mortgage allows Angie to remain in her home for the remainder of her life. If there is any money remaining in the monetary pool (currently at $29,366) it would go to her heirs. Her heirs have one year after Angie passes on to unload the furniture and let the mortgage company have the house. Or they can purchase the house from the mortgage company.

Angie gets around okay, but is no longer driving. The reason she is not driving is because her car was totaled. She had lent her car to her boarder and he totaled it. She has not purchased a new one.

For a while Angie had back problems. It took three injections of a corticosteroid to relieve the pain. Hopefully it will not return. Meanwhile, Angie does have some pain from a Sciatic nerve in her leg. It is bearable, but annoying. And sometimes it is downright painful.

Next month, Angie will be taking her first of two procedures to relieve her cataracts, one procedure for each eye. She had two choices of procedure. She could choose the more expensive one that is not covered by Medicare. It costs $3,890. Or she could choose the basic procedure that is partially covered by Medicare.

She chose the basic procedure. It will cost $707.72 for each eye. After Medicare, she will be out a total of $800.00. She will draw this from her reverse mortgage fund. The more expensive procedure would have eliminated the need for glasses. However, Angie is used to wearing glasses and does not feel this is a problem.

At the present time, Angie needs a new gas stove and wall mounted oven unit. She is making do at present. Pricing these units at the nearby superstore came to just over $1,300. She obtains meals on wheels and uses her microwave. She also needs her two window units reinstalled for the summer season.

Angie also has COPD. There is an expensive procedure that helps lung patients with COPD. This procedure costs $8,000 for the first procedure and an additional $5,000 for the second trip. At some time Angie may have to have this procedure done. It takes 3 days each session.

Angie also has a ripped tendon that she is living with. At some point she may have to have this repaired. It gives her pain in her shoulder and down her arm.

Angie has a cheerful and optimistic disposition. She enjoys anyone she is associated with. They also enjoy talking with her. She has a keen sense of humor and is a giving person.

Lifelong Monetary Plan

For most of Angie's and her husband's life they were working hard and planning to someday purchase a house, They did finally after over 30 years purchase a house. It was sad that Angie's husband died shortly after the purchase.

Angie's lifelong monetary plan was to work hard and take good care of her children. Wayne was a good provider and worked two jobs at times to support the family. Their kids did not want. They had a travel trailer that they towed on vacations. They lived most of their life in a townhouse.

Plan for the Future

Angie's plan for the future is to improve physically. She feels that once she has her eye surgery she can do things to improve her muscle mass. She used to do Yoga and may try this again. Now that she no longer has back problems, she believes that she can work on her muscle mass after she recovers from her eye operations.

SWOT Analysis (Strength, weaknesses, opportunities, Threats)

Strengths:

Angie's strength resides in her outlook. Financially, she just gets by, but she owns her own home. She has no mortgage. She lives frugally and has help from relatives and friends. Plus she has a small amount to draw from her reverse mortgage.

Weaknesses:

Angie's main weakness is the potential for her almost $30,000 stipend to run out. Medical costs are skyrocketing and Medicare does not cover everything. Also, her age may eventually, as it does with everyone, make it impossible for her to take total care of herself.

Opportunities:

Angie's main opportunities will lie in her relationship with relatives and friends. Angie believes that once she recovers from her cataract operation that she will be able to improve her overall physical condition.

Threats:

Like anyone in their late seventies, Angie has medical threats. Her reverse mortgage stipend could also eventually run out and leave Angie with nothing to fall back on. Angie's main concern is that she could die alone. No one would even know she had died for several days. She worries about her dogs having food and water if this did happen.

Civic Activities

Certainly taking in Fen, adopting him, and raising him as a son was major. Angie should certainly be proud of this. In addition Angie was a cub scout den mother all the time her boys were in cub scouts. When they became boy scouts her husband took over and led the scouts. She was also a volunteer for the American Indian Center.

Regrets

Angie listed several regrets. They are not necessarily in order of importance as follows:

1. She wished that she had kept a lifelong journal of what she and her family did.
2. She would have liked to continue with her Yoga exercises.

3. She wished that she had been better able to help her children with their homework.
4. She wished that she had taken more home movies and more records of her children's growth.
5. She also wished that she could have been stronger financially to help her aging parents.

Health

Angie is 5'7" and slender. At this point in time, Angie has several health issues. None of them are debilitating. She has mildly high blood pressure, a torn ligament in her arm, cataracts (scheduled for operation), an annoying Sciatic nerve, and COPD.

She believes that she can improve her health. She did Yoga for many years and may try doing some of these moves as she starts to feel better. She knows to be careful so that her back pain does not return.

She has been told that she can't bend down for some time after her cataract surgery. One of the questions she has for her doctor is how long must she not bend down.

Name	Age	Education	Financial Strength	Health	Age Last Worked	Plan Strength
Larry	76	Coll. Eq.	Solid	Good	66 yrs	Fair

Larry is a 76 year old male with solid financial strength. He is not rich, but he is living frugally in a 1600 sq. ft. condominium that is one part of a fourplex. This condo is in North Carolina. His monthly home owner's condo fee covers the outside lawn and maintenance. His monthly income added to his yearly draws from two IRA accounts will carry him for the rest of his life.

Larry and his wife Regina have been married for 53 years and are both in good health. Larry takes a mild blood pressure medicine. His blood pressure is fine at 140/75. He takes no other medicine and has no other issues.

Larry and his wife lived in Alabama and Mississippi the early part of their lives. They spent the last 51 years in Mobile, Alabama except for a two year stent in Birmingham. However, they just this year followed their son's and grandson's family to North Carolina and as mentioned purchased a condominium there.

Larry did not go to college after high school. He was an average student. School was marginally important. He had miscellaneous jobs after high school such as carpenter's assistant. But in the late 1960's he started a job with a Paper Mill in Mobile. This was the beginning of a fine career.

After working for several years at the paper mill, Larry joined an engineering firm in Birmingham, Al. He and his wife moved to Birmingham for two years. After two years, Larry's wife, Regina, found Larry a job back in Mobile with another engineering firm.

From the time Larry joined this firm, it started downsizing. When Larry was the last engineer at this company, he decided to jump ship. One of his close friends worked for a controls instrumentation company. He talked Larry into joining his company as a salesman. This was the beginning of a lengthy sales career for Larry in the controls instrumentation field.

When Larry moved back to Mobile, he and his wife bought a modest house on the outskirts of Mobile, Alabama. They lived in this home until his retirement from industry at the age of 66.

At age 66 Larry and his wife moved to Mobile proper. They bought a home. Shortly after purchasing this home, they decided to build their "dream home". Larry had always wanted a home with a walk out basement. That is, one of the 4 walls opening to the outside.

Larry and Regina have two married children (a boy and a girl) and three grandchildren. They moved last year to follow their son's transfer to North Carolina. Their grandson also now lives nearby in North Carolina and works as a minister's assistant. His wife is a missionary and works for a women's rights group.

Situation at Age 67

At the age of 67 Larry had been retired from working for one year. He was in the process of building his and his wife's dream house. Larry decided to be his own builder. He researched thoroughly all aspects of building. Financially at this point in his life, Larry had several sources of income as follows:

```
Social S. Larry  -- $ 28,000
Social S. wife       14,000
Pension              14,000
Two annuities        As needed and as required by law at 70 1/2
         Total   $ 56,000
```

At this point Larry had been happily married for 43 years and this marriage as mentioned had produced a son and a daughter.

Larry had used an on line software program to design the building of his new home. He decided to build a cement house. Concrete home plans have numerous structural and sustainable benefits including greater wind resistance, low maintenance, and greater insulation values. Some homes can also be poured in place. Larry's home used insulated concrete forms. Larry was his own builder.

Larry had two 401(k)'s that he had contributed to the two companies that he worked for over the years. He had accumulated a good deal of money over the years. He even put all his pay raises into 401(k's) beyond the tax free amount allowed.

When he retired, he converted these two 401(k)'s to IRA's. By law he is required to remove a certain amount each year after reaching 70 ½.   This is also true of a workplace 401(k). However if you have a Roth IRA, you are exempt from this rule and your Roth IRA earnings are tax free. You may take out this money with no taxes applied.

The amount that Larry would have to remove at age 70 1/2 is calculated by dividing his expected years remaining of life into the amount of money in the IRA. This will be approximately $20,000. The minimum tax would be 20%.

For example, at age 70 his life expectancy is 17 years (IRS publication 590-B).   So if he has $85,000 in one of his two traditional IRA's, then he would have to take out $85,000/17 or $5,000 for that year. At age 80 one's life expectancy is 10.2 years. So if one had $30,600 left in an IRA, then his required take out for that year would be $30,600/10.2 or $3,000. For every dollar below $3,000 one would have to pay fifty percent or 50 cents in income tax for each dollar below $3,000.

Physically Larry was in good shape. He loved playing golf and had a golfing family of friends. He played several times per week. He enjoyed his family and friends. He was active in the church. Plus now his house construction was taking up much of his time. As his own builder, he had to deal with subs. He decided to purchase the materials and use the subs strictly for their labor.

History Leading to Retirement

Larry was born in 1941 to farm parents living in South Central, Mississippi. His father farmed 40 acres by mule and plow. He also went down to New Orleans and worked in the ship yard there to supplement the family income.

Larry remembers the farm house well. There were cracks in the wood floor between planks. Larry's dog would spend time under the house. Larry could actually talk to his dog through the spaces between the planks.

Larry's father saved enough to start a furniture store. He had this store for 5 years, but was too soft hearted. He granted too much credit and went out of business.

Larry's father then moved the family to Louisiana where his father worked for a boiler maker. The family then moved to

North Carolina and then to Tennessee for work. When Larry was 15 his family finally settled in Mobile, Alabama.

When Larry was in high school he belonged to boy scouts. He made almost all his merit badges and became a first class scout. He was one step away from Eagle Scout.

Larry did not go to college after high school. He was an average student, but enjoyed school and as mentioned was a boy scout. After high school, he had several jobs for several years. He worked in carpentry and in the building trades. But in the late 1960's he started a job with one of the paper mills in Mobile. This was the beginning of a long and a fine career. In 1962 Larry made his most important life decision. He married Regina.

At the paper mill Larry took several tests and ended up in the instrumentation department. This was considered a prestigious job in the paper industry. Larry kept advancing in the department. He took many courses in instrumentation and electrical maintenance.

At the same time, Larry took college courses in math and science. He was getting both educational and practical experience. One of his courses was in drafting and design. He became an excellent designer. A Birmingham Engineering firm was looking for people with Larry's skill set. So Larry was hired by them and given a design engineering position.

During the time that Larry worked for this Birmingham Engineering firm, he gained practical experience in design engineering and in plant start-ups. Also during this time, Larry's wife was interested in moving back to Mobile to be near family. She actually found a similar job for Larry working with another engineering firm.

Larry did very well with this Mobile engineering firm. He started as an engineer and moved up to being the head of the instrument department. He had eight engineers working for him. While Larry was doing well, the company started to go downhill financially. It kept reducing staff until it was just the office manager and Larry.

Fortunately a friend and business associate of Larry's had been trying to influence him into going into sales with his industrial instrument control company. Although Larry was nervous about the idea of sales, he made the decision to jump a sinking ship and join his friend's instrument company.

Larry had a major advantage going for him in changing to a sales career. He had been heavily involved with local instrument societies. One of these was an instrumentation and communication society in the electrical engineering field.

Larry's friend was the district manager for the Mobile region and Larry would be working for him. The district manager had just sold a major project to Degussa Chemical and wished to hire another salesman to grow the business even more.

As they were heading east across Mobile Bay making an early sales trip Larry's new boss said "you know Larry that this is the greatest job in the world". He elaborated by stating "You get paid to see your friends".

This was absolutely true for Larry. He had been so involved through these instrument societies. He had developed so many friends from all the industries around Mobile that selling truly was "seeing your friends".

Larry learned a great deal travelling with his new boss. It was a time in industry where new hires were trained thoroughly. In addition to personal attention, Larry went through a 9 week factory training up North. Larry quickly adapted in his transition from engineering to sales. He remained in sales for almost 4 decades before retiring at the age of 66.

Larry remained with this industrial Instrumentation and Controls Company until 1992. During this time period, Larry had many sales successes. His biggest was a 4 million dollar job with a major paper mill along the Gulf Coast.

This paper mill had been purchasing their control and instrumentation from a competitor that was firmly entrenched in this mill. Larry still visited his friends in this mill even though they had not bought anything from his company.

One day while visiting one of his friends at the mill, he had an opportunity to help the head of engineering for the mill. The manager needed some instrumentation design engineering. Since Larry's forte was design engineering, Larry helped out by doing some quick work for this engineering manager.

A few weeks later, it so happened that this mill needed to be able to record environmental information. This was newly required by the Environmental Protection Agency. The mill needed it right away. Larry's competitor was on vacation for two weeks. So the mill gave Larry the opportunity to get this recording instrumentation within a three day period.

Fortunately the district office that Larry's Mobile office fell under was able to help. They started working around the clock for two days. Larry drove to their headquarters, picked up the equipment and brought it to the mill in time. By now Larry was a hero and slated for more business at the Gulf Coast mill.

The corporate vice president of all engineering for the paper mills throughout the country was to visit his Gulf Coast mill. He specifically wanted to meet with Larry. This was an honor and Larry remembers it as an interview more than a meeting. What Larry didn't know was that this mill was slated for a major expansion.

Shortly before the major expansion was announced this same corporate engineering vice president travelled to look at a computer control system at another mill. This system was manufactured by Larry's competition. This was the same competitor that had been getting all the business prior to Larry.

Travelling with the corporate vice president was a member of the engineering group at the Gulf Coast mill. They looked at the competitor system and it was a solid system. However on the way back the corporate engineer asked the Gulf States mill engineer for his opinion. He gave his opinion that Larry should get the job. So Larry got a $4 million dollar order for this new expansion.

Most of Larry's company's orders were under $50,000. So a $4 million dollar order was a mega order. Larry became a hero in his company and was eventually promoted to manage the Mobile, Al. office.

During his career with this company they instituted a 401(k) program. Larry who had been frugal all his life joined the program and also put money into the 401(k) above the amount that was tax free. This was Larry's savings account.

Larry had purchased a modest house not too far from the paper mill early in his career. He was only paying slightly over $100 per month. He lived in this house until he retired at age 66. Thus Larry had little outgo and was wise to save as much as he could in his 401(k). Larry's wife was a stay at home mother.

Larry and Regina had two children, a boy and then a girl. Both did well in life and both provided Larry and Regina with grandchildren. One of Larry's grandchildren would stay with Larry while his parents worked. He did this for most of his life. Thus Larry and Regina were not only close to their children, but close, especially to this grandson.

Shortly after Larry had been promoted to managing the office, he was demoted back to salesman. His company called to assure him that this was not to be construed negatively by Larry.

Then a few months later they promoted him back. This promoting and demoting and then promoting again occurred five times. However, the last time they contacted Larry they laid him off. The company had run into serious financial problems.

At the same time that Larry's company was having financial difficulties his old competitor from the Gulf Coast mill was making great strides. They had developed a new and modern computer control system that had advanced features. It also lacked some features that other competitors had. It depended on the salesman to accentuate the good features and downplay the not so good.

Shortly after being laid off, one of the senior technical people at the Gulf Coast Mill contacted the division manager, Joe, of Larry's old competitor. At this time this competitor no longer had any equipment in this mill. This mill had two competitors, one of which was Larry's previous company.

The senior technical mill person told Joe that he would consider it a personal favor if Joe could hire Larry. Joe already knew Larry in passing. Joe had worked with a company years ago that supplied products that were not in competition with Larry. In fact once or twice they both took the customers to lunch and split the bill. Now Joe worked for a major competitor of Larry's old company.

Joe had the ability to hire Larry and move some accounts to make a decent territory for Larry. The first account after being hired that they went after was the Gulf Coast paper mill that Larry had done so will with. They double teamed it. They were successful in taking the business away from the two current competitors. It took several years, but they did it.

Meanwhile, they were successful in bringing in other accounts and growing the business. However, things change. After Larry had been with this new company for 10 years, the company started sliding backwards financially. It had undergone several buyouts by other companies and had changed its name.

After working for this company for 13 years Larry's manager was laid off. Larry still had a job. But business was going downhill. Larry managed to be the last one standing in the Mobile territory. It was no longer fun. Larry clearly saw the writing on the wall and decided to retire at age 66. It was time.

Both Larry and Joe had had long careers in the Control and Instrumentation business. They had both started before computers were introduced to the products they carried. They carried measuring devices, valves, flow measuring devices, weight measuring devices, motors, and temperature, etc. They were part of the introduction to industrial computers utilizing their products.

Although Larry retired at age 66 from industry, Joe continued on after he was laid off at age 62. He went into sales for industrial integrators of all control products. He was no longer tied to a specific product. He could sell the services to install and engineer all or any products on the market. Joe remained working until he retired from this new discipline in his middle 70's.

They both saw the industry explode with high volume sales and then plummet as factories closed. Sales also plummet over time because these systems lasted longer and longer.

They saw these sales continue down as people were expected in these remaining factories to do more with less. Larry had been one of the last remaining people in several companies that he had worked for. He had enjoyed working with the friends that he had developed in his work. Now it was time for Larry to enjoy life without work.

Retirement Years (Beyond 67)

Larry had been frugal all his life. He lived in the same house that he and his wife bought in their early years. He wasn't rich, but because of his frugality and saving regimen was well off. Upon retirement he converted his two 401(k)'s to traditional IRA accounts. When he started drawing from these at 70 ½ it amounted to about $20,000 per year.

The traditional IRA account contributions like Larry's are taxed on both federal and state tax returns on the year you make the withdrawal. Withdrawals in retirement or at any time are taxed as ordinary income tax rates.

Larry was able to roll over to an IRA with no tax penalty. Then as he withdraws he must pay taxes at the normal tax rates for his income. However, since Larry is no longer making a large income his tax rate is lower when he does take it out. As noted earlier the amount that Larry would have to remove at age 70 1/2 and each year thereafter is calculated by dividing his expected years remaining of life into the amount of money in the IRA. The life expectancy chart and information on IRA's as mentioned earlier can be found in IRS publication 590-B.

Right after retirement at 67, Larry moved from his Alabama home of 35 years to a house in Mobile proper. His old house had been seriously flooded due to hurricane Katrina. Fortunately he had flood insurance.

Once in Mobile, Larry began designing his dream home. He used a software package called Punch! Software. Punch! allows you to design your home plans from many angles. You can move rooms around and view your plan in many dimensions. It is like having your own architect.

Once Larry was finished with his plan, he began subcontracting the work. He had to do quite a bit of research. He decided early on to purchase all materials direct and only use subs for labor. The Punch! Software provided a materials list. The finished home would have a walk out basement and be 3500 square feet in living area.

Unfortunately, Larry did the same thing as Jeffrey and many others that built their dream house. They overbuilt for the area. Thus a house that may have cost $450,000 would only sell for $400,000. Also a basement with only one outside wall does not carry the appraisal of an above ground level.

Larry lived in this house until he was 76. He enjoyed golfing with his golfing buddies that he had for over 30 years. He was active and happy. He and Regina enjoyed their church, relatives, and friends.

Then at about the age of 75 both his son and his son's wife moved to North Carolina for job opportunity. At about the same time Larry's grandson also moved to North Carolina.

While Larry had lived frugally most of his life, building his dream house was a departure from living frugally. He enjoyed this new life style for about 8 years. Then he and his wife decided to follow their children to North Carolina and live there. They sold their home in Mobile taking a $50,000 loss. But they were happy to be moving to be with their family.

They were also happy to downsize from a 3500 square foot house to a 1600 square foot condominium. They were extremely fortunate in that the purchasers of their house also needed furniture. They were moving from a rental in Italy. So Larry and Regina were able to sell them their furniture. The only thing Larry misses is his golfing family community. He will have to develop a new golfing group. In the meantime he is enjoying just doing nothing.

Lifelong Monetary Plan

Larry was at the head of his class with regards to preparing for retirement. He had started savings from very early in life. He lived frugally virtually his whole life. He continued savings until retirement. And even in retirement at age 76 he was again saving by living frugally.

Plan for the Future

Larry plans to develop a golfing group. He will never be able to replace the long-time friends that he had in Mobile. Larry also needs to regain his stamina for playing as many holes as he was used to in Mobile. Right now he and Regina are just getting acclimated to their new setting. Their real plan will be to develop a plan.

However, they do plan at some time to travel out west. They will not fly, but they will drive. For now Larry is going to enjoy not having anything to specifically do.

SWOT Analysis

Strengths:

Larry's strength comes from his home life and family. He has always had stability in family and friends. Financially, Larry is set for the rest of his life. His health is good and so is his wife's. Larry and Regina are among the very fortunate retirees.

Weaknesses:

Like any retirees Larry and Regina are getting to an age when health could become an issue. Being in a new environment brings stresses of its own. It also brings new life. It will depend on how Larry and Regina approach their new environment.

Opportunities:

Larry's main opportunity comes from his financial strength. He will have disposable income left over each month. He and Regina plan to do some travelling. They have a whole new life ahead of them.

Threats:

There are no immediate threats in Larry's and Regina's life. Like all retirees they are facing the perils of approaching age, but this will hopefully not rear its ugly head for some time.

Civic Activities

Larry was always a joiner. And as a joiner in civic activities he was usually asked to be part of the governing body. He was president of one of the instrument societies. He also was active in the Technical Association of the Pulp and Paper Industry (TAPPI).

Larry has always been active in church groups. He belonged for many years to a men's group at Church. He was the oldest member with the longest longevity. He helped build a new Sanctuary.

Beyond civic activities, Larry was always encouraging people as part of his personality. Larry would help anyone that needed help at any time. You could always rely on Larry. As a matter of fact, Larry suggested that I put together a check list for people moving from one location to another as part of this book.

Since I have moved 14 times in my life, I felt that I could certainly put this together. I then ran it by Larry since he had just moved from Alabama to North Carolina. So attached in Exhibit 1 is a check list for those of you who are preparing for or are in the middle of a move.

Regrets

Larry regrets not having been more of a Christian. He was always a solid Christian, but over the past 10 years he has experienced an increased joy and peace in his Christian beliefs. As giving as Larry has always been he wished that he had been more giving in his earlier years. So this is his number one regret. That he had been more giving earlier even though he was more giving by far than the majority of people that I know.

Health Issues

Larry has no health issues nor does his wife. Larry does need to do more exercise now that he is not playing as much golf as he used to.

Chapter 8
(Steve)

Name	Age	Education	Financial Strength	Health	Age Last Worked	Plan Strength
Steve	84	College	Moderate	Fair	66 yrs	Fair

As can be seen above, Steve is an 84 year old man who worked until he was 66 and then retired. Steve was born and raised in Vancouver, Washington. His father worked at the paper mill. Steve's family could trace its origins back to the incorporation of Vancouver in the late 1850's.

Steve's family originally had a large piece of land on the outskirts of Vancouver. Over the years they had sold off most of the land and today have only 5 acres left where his parents lived. Steve had an unremarkable high school career. He tried out for football in the 10th grade, but did not do well. He could run fast, but was clumsy and did not really like the long training hours. He did not finish out the season.

Steve played intramural sports, baseball and basketball. He also made the tennis team his senior year. His parents agreed to pay the first two years of each of their three children's college career. Steve had two older sisters and they had both made it through all four years by going to school at night. They were both nurses.

Steve took business courses as his major and he minored in math. It took him 6 years to get through. He worked part time at several jobs and was able to work at the paper mill in the summers because of his father's position at the mill. His father was a millwright at the mill. Steve was a paper machine attendant. He mostly cleaned up the waste paper.

When he graduated he obtained a job in the accounting department at the mill. He did not like the work, but he met his future wife in the accounting department. She was a clerical person in the accounting department.

His wife was originally from Houston, Texas. After a few years, Steve obtained a job in Houston working for a chemical plant as an assistant in the purchasing department. Steve's wife, Linette thought that she would be happy living back in her home state. But after 3 children were born she was ready to move on to any place Steve wanted to go. Now Steve and his wife had two girls and a son, just like his parents had. All three children were under 7 when Steve decided to change careers. He lucked out and found a position as a salesman working for a paper mill supplier in Mobile, Alabama.

Steve was hired because of his knowledge of the wet end of a paper machine. He had worked summers on the machines. It was odd that he did obtain this job because this company usually hired people who had already sold products to paper mills.

So Steve moved his family to Mobile, Alabama and purchased a house in a subdivision called Amberly Subdivision. It was a modest house and reasonably priced. He had made a profit on his house sale in Houston. He sold his Houston house the first week-end on the market.

Steve's sales career was marginal at best. After 3 years he moved back to his home in Vancouver. His parents had recently died. He moved into their old house and worked out an arrangement with his two sisters who both still lived in parts of the Northwest.

Steve was able to obtain a job at his old paper mill in the purchasing department. After several years he became the purchasing manager of the department. He retired from this job at the mill. Steve fixed up his parents place. He played golf and was active in city politics. He ran for political office, but did not succeed.

Steve decided to use his 10 acres to organic farm. He did this for a while until he sold 5 acres to a developer. Steve has COPD and heart trouble. He is now at 84 somewhat sedentary. He still is able to walk, but his knees bother him if he walks too far. He still drives. They like to go to the other Vancouver in Canada. They also travel down the coast. He and his wife take short trips for vacation. She does most of the driving.

Situation at Age 67

At age 67 Steve had been finished with his job for almost one year. He was collecting social security. Linette had worked as an accounting assistant for a company that had a pension program. She collected $540 per month in retirement. They had no other source of monthly income. He did have a healthy 401(k) that had $180,000 in it.

Steve also had a savings account with $80,000 which mostly came from the sale of half of his land. He had used some of the money from the sale to help his three children and pay off his mortgage. He had sold this land almost 10 years ago. It took several years before the developer began building homes. So between he and his wife their yearly income from social security and Linette's pension was:

```
Social S. Steve        --          $ 26,800
Social S. Linette                    13,400
Pension for Linette                   6,480
                        Total     $ 46,680
```

Steve and Linette had no mortgage. Their house was clear and had been renovated over the years. They had bought out Steve's sister's share. Their children were long gone. They visited with them often. Between the three children they had six grandchildren. Over the years the grandchildren had all enjoyed visiting Steve's "farm".

Steve and Linette had fun farmed over the years. They mostly grew organic vegetables, herbs, and watermelons. They made a few thousand dollars by selling directly to local residents. They even had some chickens and a goat. But all this was gone. It disappeared when they sold off their land to a developer several years ago.

The developer had put in paved roads and started building and selling middle range houses for the spreading suburbanites that were now reaching out towards Steve and Linette's area. The houses were starting to sell.

Steve had been contacted to sell another 3 acres to the developer. Steve felt he could get a better price than he did last time. They had come back to Steve with two offers, which he smartly refused. The last time, they offered to purchase his entire property at a significant price and build him a fine home at no cost. It was an attractive offer. He had not yet responded.

Steve's older sister was dead now. His next oldest was in good shape. Steve was reluctant to sell the old homestead. He asked his sister if she would mind. She said it was his property now and he could do what he wanted with it. So Steve was thinking of taking their latest offer. The farmhouse, although renovated over the years, was not worth much in its own right.

Steve and Linette had purchased a travel trailer that they hitched to their F-150. They knew most of the camp areas. Since they had retired from active work they hit the roads quite often now. Both Steve and Linette were in good physical shape. So life was good for them.

At the beginning of the new Millennia, they were reasonably secure financially. They did not have a large income, but it was enough for now. Plus they had a small reserve that they could draw from if necessary. They did not take any medicines and relied solely on Medicare parts A and B.

History Leading to Retirement

Steve was born in 1933 and raised on the outskirts of Vancouver, Washington. When Steve grew up his parents had 20 acres. This was down from the original 80 acres that their forbearers owned. The land had been periodically sold off to keep the family going. In fact, during Steve's lifetime, his father sold off 10 acres.

Steve's father was a millwright at the paper mill. His mother was a homemaker. Steve had two older sisters that treated Steve like their own child. He was 6 and 4 years younger than his sisters. Since they were not that close to neighbors, Steve grew up in his early years playing with his sisters. He did however, play early sports in grade school.

Steve grew into a handsome teenager. By the time he was 14 he was his final height of 5'10'' and weighed 150 pounds. Steve played intramural baseball and basketball through his 4 years of high school. He was also popular with the girls.

Scholastically Steve was a B student. School came easy to him. This was partially because his sisters helped him with homework. He took math through trigonometry and excelled in math.

Steve lived 10 miles from school and took his bicycle to school every day. He never missed a day of school for illness. In the 10th grade he tried out for the football team. Steve was a fast sprinter, but he was clumsy and messed up plays. He played in the backfield. After a month, Steve dropped out of football. He didn't like the long hours of practice.

Steve had an aunt who was an exceptional piano player. She played at the church every Sunday. One day when Steve was 6 and visiting his aunt he showed an interest and talent for the piano. So his aunt started tutoring Steve in the piano. He did not have a piano at home so he could only practice on his aunt's piano. When Steve was in the 6ᵗʰ grade his aunt died. She willed the piano to Steve.

So at the age of 10 Steve now could practice as much as he wanted. He had gained the rudiments of piano and had an excellent ear. He had also inherited a great deal of sheet music from his aunt.

By the time he was in the 10ᵗʰ grade, Steve was so good at the piano that he and 3 others formed a band. They were so good that they performed at weddings and dances. They even got paid. Steve was talented, but not talented enough to really do anything truly professionally.

When Steve was ready for college his two sisters had just completed nursing programs. Their parents had paid for the first two years of tuition and were willing to do the same for Steve. He went to college locally and made income playing the piano in his band and working summers in the paper mill.

His last two years of college took him 4 years to complete. This was partly because of money and partly because Steve enjoyed the party life. Steve majored in business and minored in math. He was good in math and did very well. His business courses were C and C+ grade. He did get A's in all his accounting courses.

His first job out of college was as an accounting assistant at the paper mill where he had worked summers. The work was boring, but he met an accounting clerk there that he instantly knew was the one for him. She apparently felt the same way because she went everywhere Steve wanted to go. Her name was Linette. She was pretty and slim and had a great sense of humor. She and Steve married after 8 months of dating.

Linette and Steve started a family within the first year of marriage. They had a boy. Yet it was 5 years before they had their next two children who were identical twin girls. All their children were healthy.

Right after their son was born, Steve took night classes to get his MBA. It took him 5 years, but he did well. He ended up with a 3.8 GPA.

Shortly after the twins were born, Steve had an opportunity to become the assistant purchasing manager at a chemical plant in Houston, Texas. This plant had been looking for someone with accounting, operations, and an MBA degree. Steve fit the bill.

He also had one of his wife's relatives that worked at the chemical plant pulling for him. Linette was glad to be back in Houston where she had relatives.

Steve and Linette stayed in Houston for several years until Steve was 41. Linette and Steve decided that they would like to get out of the Houston area and live along the Gulf Coast. They had been to Gulf Shores, Alabama for vacation several times. They just liked the area.

So Steve applied for jobs in both Mobile and Pensacola through a Head Hunter. He lucked out right away. A company that sold the large belts called plastic wires, felts, and dryer fabrics hired him. The plastic wires were the belts that the wet pulp from dissolving wood chips with alkaline flowed onto.

The water was drained through these porous moving belts or plastic wires. The paper was then picked up by the moving felts and dried further through pressure. The paper then went into a dryer section that contained several dryer felts that dried the paper to its final dryness. Steve sold the third group, the dryer felts.

The dryer felts that Steve sold were not the strongest product that his new company produced. The strongest product was plastic wires that were sold for the wet end of the machine where the wet stock poured out from a "head box". Steve decided to team with the plastic wire salesman in his company.

All three products had a salesman that sold those products exclusively. However, they all three called on the same customers in the mill. So, once a month Steve and the plastic wire salesman would travel together.

They would entertain the customers jointly the night before going into the paper mills to sell their products. They would then after having dinner usually with the paper mill superintendent and his wife go into the mill the next morning. Sometimes they would take a large group of paper mill people out for lunch to further enhance their chances of sale.

The plastic wire salesman was the top salesman for the company. He helped Steve sell his dryer felts because of his relationship with the customers. Many times Steve would not get in to see the customer on his own. But by travelling with the plastic wire salesman he was able to see and sell some product.

In the evenings both Steve and the wire salesman, Jake, would go to a local bar. This was during the 70's when most places in the evening had dance floors and served liquor along with the dancing.

Steve and Jake, although married, joined in with the dancing. Jake was more conservative in his drinking. Many times they would stay at motels that had both dancing and drinking right on the premises. Jake would usually leave and go to his room or have Steve take him back to the motel they were staying at by 11:00 P.M. Steve preferred to stay late.

Jake would only have two beers while Steve would drink hard liquor. Steve started drinking more and more. He also took some of his dancing partners back to his room for the night. He was having a mid-life crisis.

Jake enjoyed Steve's company and didn't mind his extended carousing. Steve was always sharp the next morning. He sometimes looked a little rough, but always made it. Jake and Steve would laugh and kid each other about their night's activities. It was the 1970's and things were morally loose.

One night that was not on their normal routine week, Jake happened to be out at a local motel night club. He saw Steve coming out of the bathroom obviously drunk. Steve made a beeline for an older woman that he was obviously with. They were both "three sheets to the wind" as the saying goes. Jake quietly left the night club.

Jake didn't see Steve for two weeks until their scheduled week together. Steve was starting to look "rough". Steve's sales had just been mediocre. But most of the dryer felt salesmen were mediocre. However, the last three months had been poor sales months for Steve.

In the car after having dinner with customers, Jake did mention that he saw Steve at the night club. Steve immediately started to cry. Jake was floored. Steve confessed that his drinking and carousing had gotten the best of him. Mixed with his crying, he said he loved his wife and kids and felt that he had let them down. He asked if he should confess his sins to his wife.

Jake didn't know what to say, but did advise Steve not to tell his wife about his carousing with other women. He suggested telling her that he had a drinking problem. He suggested asking her for help and advice. Steve said that he had no control over his actions. Steve decided right then and there to go home to his wife.

They were about 120 miles from home, but Jake took Steve home and then drove back to his motel. He didn't get back to the motel until almost 4 A.M. He had a 9:00 A.M. meeting in the mill that he was just able to make it to.

When Steve got back to his home, Linette immediately knew something was wrong. Steve started crying as he told Linette about his drinking problem. He took Jake's advice and never told her about the women he had been with.

Linette was comforting and understanding. This made Steve feel both relieved and guilty. She realized that Steve needed to "get off the road". She realized that selling was not for Steve. When she said this to him, he realized that she was absolutely correct. Steve didn't like selling and had to push himself to be reasonably good at it.

Admitting to himself that he wasn't a salesman was like a great weight being removed off his chest. Linette said that she would do whatever he wanted. The next morning it was Linette who came up with a plan.

Steve slept late. Linette was real busy while Steve slept. She had called several people and talked to them real early in the morning. When Steve came down she said that she had talked to Steve's two sisters.

They had agreed that Steve could have the family farm outside Vancouver that had been sitting empty since their parent's death. They said that Steve could pay them monthly until their shares were paid up. They would get an appraisal and then settle on a payment schedule.

Further Linette had called one of her friends at the paper mill where they had both worked. She found out that the mill was looking for a new purchasing manager. The previous manager had been just caught taking money from vendors. Steve could apply for this job. This didn't mean he would get it, but he stood a good chance.

Steve was ecstatic. He liked the mill and he had enjoyed his previous purchasing job. He should never have gone into sales. Steve had two weeks' vacation coming. So they gave their Mobile, Alabama home to an agent. They sold as much of their possessions as they could and moved back to Washington State.

Steve called his old mill and talked to the mill manager. He set up an interview two weeks ahead. So he and Linette and the kids got a large U-Haul trailer and hitched it to their car. They had North American move the rest of their possessions.

They made it to Vancouver in 8 days. They stopped along the way to sight see at the Grand Canyon and at Yellowstone. The kids loved missing school for a week. Steve eventually got the purchasing manager's job.

The old farmhouse was in rough condition, but Steve and Linette and their children adored the place. In time they would fix it up and modernize it as much as possible. Steve sold 5 of the 10 acres to help pay his sisters and fix up the place.

Until he sold off the 5 acres, Linette spearheaded an organic garden of vegetables, herbs, spices, and watermelons. She found local families that she contracted with for her produce. She hired some local workers and she actually made a small profit.

At the age of 66, Steve decided he had worked long enough and so retired. He and Linette had paid off the sisters and had no debts. Their children were grown and married. Two of them had gone to college and the third, the oldest girl, was in California working in Hollywood. She was what was called a "bit" player. She also did commercials. She was very pretty.

Steve had had several offers to sell his remaining five acres and the farmhouse itself. He resisted all offers and remained in the house.

Retirement Years

After retirement both Steve's and Linette's health was good. They had the camper and took many trips across the country. They knew the camp sites. Many times they would meet up with people they had met in the past. They had a long list of these people. They would call them up to see if they could join their plans together and meet at specific camp sites.

At 75 Steve started having heart problems. At first it was just shortness of breath, but he had to have several operations. He was doing okay, but would never have his old energy.

Lifelong Monetary Plan

Steve did not have a lifelong monetary plan. He did work towards paying off his sisters and fixing up his farm and acreage. He did not think about retiring until he was no longer able to keep his interest in his purchasing manager's job. He and Linette were relatively frugal.

They took their social security and Linette's small pension and just lived on this amount of money plus their 401(k) withdrawals each year. They had sold half of their property and put this money towards paying off the sisters and the rest went into a small savings which they didn't touch until late in life when inflation caught up with them.

Plan for the Future

Steve and Linette's plan for the future is to strongly consider selling their property and moving into a development home. The developer who had purchased earlier property had offered to buy the rest of Steve's property some time ago. He had also offered to build them a new home in the development. Based on current outgo and current income it would likely be necessary to sell the remaining property.

The problem that Steve and Linette had was where to live between selling their property and moving into a newly built home. Steve figured they could remain in the farmhouse while the developer built on the north end of his property. Then they could move in and the developer could bulldoze the farmhouse and continue his development.

Steve and Linette really didn't have much choice. They now planned to contact the developer and see if he was still interested in their property. They guessed that he would be, but Steve and Linette had rebuffed him so many times that they were unsure. They thought of contacting other developers and builders to see who would give them the best deal. At any rate their plan was to reluctantly sell their remaining piece of property.

SWOT Analysis

Strengths:

Steve's strength comes from his stable family environment namely his wife Linette. He never did tell her about his carousing. He never again touched liquor. His other strength comes from his family farm that had added additional money to his full time job. And his third strength came from his steady job with the paper mill.

Weakness:

Steve's weakness comes from inflation and health. At age 84 his health is starting to deteriorate. He can no longer do the things he used to. He cannot mow the grass and he can't go for walks like he used to. He sits too much. Plus he may have to have a pig valve in his heart. He takes medicine for his heart. He had a mild heart attack 5 years ago.

Opportunities:

The sale of his farm represents an opportunity to have enough money to last Steve the rest of his life. He won't be rich, but he will no longer have to stress over the unexpected repair bills or medical issues.

Threats:

Steve's biggest threat is his health. The heart attack five years ago left him week. He never fully recovered back to his old self. Also his doctors believe that he is a candidate for a pig valve. Steve's symptoms are that he is tired and short winded a good part of the time.

He no longer had the energy to do the things he would like. He and Linette have talked about a vacation without driving. They plan to fly next time. The money from the sale of the farm would permit this kind of entertainment.

Civic Activities

Steve was never a volunteer outside of his work activities. As purchasing manager he was involved in civic activities through the company. He never shirked a civic activity, but never initiated one either.

Regrets

Steve's biggest regret is having "cheated" on Linette. He still is bothered by this even after all these years. He has always been a good husband except for this one period of time in his life. He could blame it on the drinking, but he still knew it was wrong. He will take this bad feeling to his grave. He has always loved

Linette. He wonders how he could ever have slipped like this. There are days that he doesn't think about it, but it crops up at the oddest moments.

Health Issues

As mentioned, Steve's health has deteriorated. Fortunately there are no mental disorders like Alzheimer's. Steve is as sharp as he always has been.   His heart is his main worry. His doctor has him on medicine. His doctor feels that at some point he will have to have an operation to replace his heart valve with a pig's valve. Steve hates the idea of another operation.

Name	Age	Education	Financial Strength	Health	Age Last Worked	Plan Strength
Lottie	73	RN	Moderate	Fair	65 yrs	Good

As can be seen by the chart above, Lottie is a 73 year old woman. She is now retired and has fair health. She has high blood pressure and mild COPD.   Lottie has been married twice and divorced twice. Her first marriage lasted 9 years and her second lasted 22 years. She is still an active person with a positive and friendly outgoing personality.

Lottie has a significant other who is younger (20 years) than herself. Her significant other (Joe) has offered marriage, but Lottie feels that having gone through two divorces she is not marriage material. Yet they have lived together successfully for the past 18 years. They share expenses and enjoy life together.

Lottie was born and raised in Peekskill, New York. Her parents had a traditional marriage and remained together until the death of Lottie's mother at age 75. Lottie has one sister six years younger than herself.

Lottie's mother was a loving woman. She always looked after Lottie and her sister in a motherly fashion. She would take them to picnics, to the beach, and other play areas. She insisted that they go as a family to their grandmother's house at least one Sunday per month.   Lottie's father's sister and her family also made the Sunday visit. Lottie and her sister matched up in age with their two boy cousins so that these Sunday's were always special to Lottie and her cousins.

Lottie's mother initiated visits with her sister in law and the two cousins that matched in age with her children. They would go on picnics, to the beach, and to other children's gatherings.

Even though Lottie's father was strict and not the best Dad in the world he did provide the family with a nice house and stable life style. Lottie did okay in high school. But her senior year she became pregnant with her first of two children. The first child born to Lottie and her husband was born shortly after high school graduation.

Since Lottie's father did not believe in education, Lottie did not go to college. Plus she now had a husband and daughter shortly after high school graduation

During her second marriage, Lottie went back to school and obtained an RN degree. She worked as a nurse at a hospital for over 20 years. During her nursing career she worked at two different hospitals. Towards the end of her nursing career she obtained a second career as a server. She worked at two fine restaurants. One of these called Susie's was a restaurant that the governor of New York frequented.

Lottie got to serve and meet Governor Pataki who was born and raised in Peekskill. Lottie had interesting conversations with the Governor.

Just before her 67th birthday, Lottie stopped working. Her health and years of work had been enough. She wasn't in bad health, but it was just time to stop working. She and Joe lived in an apartment and then moved into her father's old house. It had been going to ruin with no one living in it. She and Joe shared expenses and fixed up the house.

Situation at Age 67

At 67 Lottie was now fully retired from work. She and her significant other, Joe, were living together in her father's old house as discussed above. Financially, Lottie was collecting her social security and sharing expenses with Joe.

Financially, Lottie had her social security and Joe's share of the costs as follows:

Social S.	$18,000
Joe's share	$18,000
Alimony	$6,000
Total	$42,000

The house was mortgage free and the taxes on the house were negligible. Lottie and Joe lived comfortably. Lottie still had money ($58,000) from the 1995 sale of the original house she and her first husband purchased for $6,000 in 1963. She had used up the money she obtained from her second divorce, but she still receives alimony.

Lottie's father was still alive at the age of 93. He was financially well off and living with his second wife in another state. At some point in time Lottie will receive a significant inheritance.

Lottie had inherited diabetes from her fraternal grandmother. Lottie is in fair physical shape other than the diabetes she inherited at age 63 and the beginnings of COPD.

At 67 Lottie has great spirit and a happy personality. She and Joe spent time with Joe's young children. Lottie also spent time with her granddaughter who lives two doors down form her. They have a great relationship. This relationship is much better than Lottie has with her own daughter.

Unfortunately Lottie's son lives in Florida. They keep up with each other by phone. Lottie is much closer to her son than her daughter.

Lottie does not keep up with her younger sister, Maggie. Her younger sister moved to Pennsylvania when Lottie was in her 30's. Maggie didn't have much to do with Lottie's side of the family and so Lottie and she don't see each other or keep in touch.

History leading to Retirement

As previously mentioned Lottie was born and grew up in Peekskill, New York. She claims her early life was totally uneventful. In school she was more into the social aspect than the educational aspect of school. She still has relationships with some of her grade school and high school friends.

Lottie preferred outside activities. When she was in high school she obtained a serving job at an exclusive resort for working business women. Lottie's father was very domineering and made her quit this job even though she truly enjoyed working there.

Growing up with a domineering father made for a very lonesome life for Lottie in her early and even into high school years.

When she was a senior in high school she became pregnant. She and her boyfriend married right after high school.

Their first child was a girl. Both her husband Harry and Lottie worked at jobs locally. Lottie obtained a job working for the county of Westchester.

By the age of 20 Lottie had a second child. This child was a boy. Lottie did not have any more children. While Lottie worked, her mother would care for the children.

Lottie and Harry were able to purchase a very cute house and seemed to have a happy relationship. But Lottie was very lonesome because Harry was gone quite a bit. After 9 years she and Harry divorced.

Lottie continued to work and kept the house. She soon met a man named Nathan. She and Nathan married and moved into the house that Lottie owned. Nathan and his family were Jewish and so Lottie became indoctrinated into the Jewish faith. Nathan was not orthodox and so it was not a major adjustment for Lottie. But she enjoyed the Jewish Religion and participated in the festivities and activities.

Nathan was doing well in his field. He trained seeing eye dogs. Together they vacationed extensively through Europe and in the U.S. They started with their honeymoon in Portugal. They travelled by rail wherever they went.

During her life with Nathan, Lottie went back to school. She obtained a bachelor's degree and an RN license. She began a 20 year career with two local hospitals.

Lottie and Nathan had a good life. They went into New York to see plays and partake of the night life in New York. They had an active life. Lottie became part of Nathan's Jewish lifestyle.

During her marriage with Nathan Dottie took up running. She would get up at 7:00 A.M. and ran 10 miles. She fell in love with running. She feels that she overdid it because she developed arthritis and had to quit running in her mid-50's.

After 15 years of marriage, Nathan was asked to take on a sales role with his seeing eye company. He then ended up travelling and thus he was gone quite a lot of the time.

Somewhere along the line in his working with training dogs for the blind he met and fell in love with a blind woman. He divorced Lottie. Lottie still had the house, but was now on her own again at age 53.

She was working two hospital jobs and then also took a job as a server for a lodge in a nearby town. At the age of 55 she left the hospital jobs that she had worked for many years.

After she retired from her RN jobs, Lottie also started a second server job with Susie's restaurant. Susie's was a famous Italian restaurant in a nearby town.

Lottie then sold her house in 1995 for $73,000 and didn't know where she was going to go and what she was going to do with the rest of her life. She was now totally independent. She no longer had a male dominating her life. She truly enjoyed her job at Susie's and so remained there for quite a while. She owned a small Harley motorcycle and cycled to work.

For the next three years, Lottie partied and just enjoyed life. After a few years she met Joe. Joe was much younger (20 years) than Lottie. Even though there was a large age difference Lottie and Joe hit it off from the moment they met. They moved in together in Lottie's apartment nearby.

Joe was divorced with young children. Lottie and Joe would take them with them to the beach, to Play Land and other appropriate places for young children.

Joe and Lottie purchased a large Harley motorbike. They travelled all over Connecticut, Massachusetts, New York, and in summer they took it to the beaches in New Jersey.

Retirement Years (Beyond 67)

Lottie fully retired from work in her mid-sixties. She and Joe moved into her father's old place when Lottie was 69. It had been empty for a while because her father and his second wife had moved. They were living on his second wife's family farm in a nearby state. Lottie and Joe took care of the house and fixed it up.

Lottie's father's wife then had a stroke that put her in a nursing home. Lottie's father wanted to come back and live in his home in Peekskill. As a matter of fact the family of his second wife demanded that Lottie immediately come and get him.

By this time he was in his mid-nineties. He was a handful to say the least. So Lottie drove the three hours to get her father.

One time her father became sick and had to go to the emergency room. He had a broken hip and this had to be operated on. When Lottie and Joe took him home after the operation their car broke down. This car was an old Buick that had been sitting in the garage of the house that she and Joe had taken over. It had been covered with so much stuff that Lottie didn't even know there was a car there.

Once she did realize it was there she started driving it. Lottie's step mother in law had to find the ownership papers because her father couldn't be bothered and didn't really want to give the car to Lottie.

Lottie and Joe did the best they could with him for six months. They just had trouble handling him. He would get up in the middle of the night and wander out into the streets. Lottie and Joe just could not control his nighttime activities.

They then put him in a nursing home and had to move him after a while to a second more expensive nursing home.

After they put her father in a nursing home, Joe and Lottie's life came back to normal. They both had arthritis in their backs and thus no longer could ride their big Harley. They purchased a Volkswagen Jetta to replace the Buick. Joe still had his old Chevy truck.

By now her father was in his late 90's and was infirm. He could not walk and so he would be more manageable. So they decided to move him back in with them. Meanwhile he had to be taken to the hospital for a bad bout with Sepsis. When he recovers Lottie and Joe will move him back with them.

Plan for the Future

With her father approaching 99, Lottie and Joe are preparing for his passing on. His health seems to be deteriorating rapidly. They have talked about what they would do when he does pass. They will take many motor trips. They will visit Lottie's son in Florida. They will travel to New England. They may go back to Prince Edward Island. Lottie truly enjoyed her vacation some time ago in Prince Edward Island.

SWOT Analysis

Strengths:

Lottie's strength lies in her positive outlook on life and her outgoing personality. While she is not rich by any stretch, she will eventually have a good inheritance from her father. While she is not close to all her relatives, she is close to her granddaughter and her son. Fortunately, her granddaughter only lives two doors down from Lottie.

Lottie also has a great relationship with her significant other. Although he wishes to marry Lottie, she is reluctant because of her two past experiences with marriage. But they share their lives and are happy.

Weaknesses:

Lottie's main weakness is her impending care for her father in her home. He is not the easiest person to deal with when he is with all his faculties. Being infirm may help with his not wandering off, but his general demeanor will make it rough on Lottie and Joe.

Opportunities:

Lottie's opportunity comes in what she will do with the rest of her life. Assuming she receives a healthy inheritance, she can plan a long comfortable life. The opportunity will be in developing a plan that makes sense and fits Lottie's life style.

Threats:

As with anyone in her 70's, health is going to be a threat. Lottie will need to follow her doctor's advice and take good care of herself. The other major threat is the impending care of her father. This could put a strain on her relationship with Joe. It could also be a major mental and physical strain on Lottie. The size of her house will make it difficult to isolate her father from Lottie's and Joe's routines.

Civic Activities

While Lottie was not specifically in any civic activities, she served people in her work capacities. As a nurse, she cared for many patients. She also became involved with the Jewish faith while she was married to Nathan.

Regrets

Lottie had to think about this for a while. At the end she said that she had no real regrets. She had a good life and did many things. She has a natural happy spirit and makes everyone she talks to feel good.

Health Issues

The only thing that slows Lottie down is her arthritis in her back. It doesn't stop her from going and coming, but she and

Joe can no longer ride their big Harley. It just sits in the garage gathering dust. She hates to sell it because of all the fine memories associated with this bike. Lottie also has mild COPD, but this does not slow her down. Her Diabetes is well controlled with pills. She is not to the point of injections yet and may never get there.

Chapter 10
Summary and Commentary

This section will look at the main issues that face retirees and provide helpful information for those either just reaching retirement or fully in retirement. It will relate these issues to the ten typical retirees in this book.

It was hard to find 10 that were totally representative. In this section we will provide the national averages for retirees. They very closely parallel the 10 retirees in this narrative. All of the ten had been married. So those who had remained single all their lives were not represented.

Interestingly there was an 11th member who could have been included. He had never married, but he spent most of his life living with a male in a homosexual relationship. His and his mate's life paralleled the married couple's lives. We also know of a heterosexual female couple who live together and their lives also paralleled the 10 married couple's lives.

In this commentary we will cover the following issues:

1. Health and Exercise   7. Downsizing
2. Financial   8. Excess Stuff
3. Plan for Future   9. Best locations for Retirees
4. Doctors   10. Moving
5. Medical   11. Reverse Mortgage
6. Family   12. Investing
        13. How do You Compare to Other Retirees?

Health and Exercise

In real estate the 3 most important words are location, location, location. In the life of a retiree, the 3 most important words are walk, walk, walk. Some may have their own exercise routine. For this reason, we almost said exercise, exercise, exercise. But we didn't for good reasons.

Sure if you have your own exercise routine and it is working for you---fine. Just keep it up. But for the majority of retirees who do not have a routine exercise then walking is truly important. You can compare walking to running, swimming, tennis or any aerobics or anaerobic, but they all have more cons than pros for retirees. The main thing is you need to be up off your butt.

Walking 5 times per week at 2-3 miles of distance is the best routine for a long life. If you add muscle training of any sort then you are golden. It doesn't have to be weight lifting. Ten pushups, laying on your back and doing the butterfly (this is recommended to prevent spine curvature), and putting your legs over the arm of a sofa or chair and then raising each with a 5-10 pound weight 20 times are the three exercises besides walking that I do and have done for most of my life.

The leg exercise had solved my knee problems while running 20 years ago. I do these religiously. I just used grey tape and taped a weight to an old running shoe. I then put on the shoe and drape my leg over the arm of a sofa in our home and lift each leg 20 times.

But before we look at the other 11 issues facing retirees, let's compare some of the issues of the ten in this book as follows:

Name	Age	Finance at age 67	Finance @ Retirement	Health	Age Last Worked*	Plan Strength
Jeff	75	130k	53k plus	Good	74.5	Good
Gloria	86	48.4k	48.4k	Fair	33	Poor
Roger	68	121.2k	62k	Good	67	Good
Mary	94	36.7	36.7	Failed	65	N.A.
Clete	98	57k	19.4k	Poor	70	Fair
Angie	79	23.2K	18.4k	Fair	60	Fair
Larry	76	57.5k	77k	Good	65	Good
Steve	84	46.7	46.7	Fair	66	Good
Lottie	73	42k	42k	Fair	65	Fair
Average	81.4	62.5	44.8			

Since we started with health, it is interesting to note that two of the three retirees that have good health routinely walk. Jeff and Roger walk in their neighborhoods. They each walk 5-6 times per week.

Larry does virtually no exercise.. He used to play golf several times per week, but since moving to North Carolina he has not played golf. He now has prostate problems (up 6 times per night) and does not feel as good as he did since moving. He had to postpone our second interview because he felt awful. I still gave him a "good" but this may have to be downgraded to fair.

There are two health issues that virtually every male has and virtually every female has. For the males it is prostate problems and for females it is hormones. Every one of our 10 retirees had and/or has these two issues.

Prostate problems as you men know first appear when you get up multiple times at night to go to the bathroom. It gets worse from there. There are a number of remedies for this problem. Each person is different and thus each person must decide with his urologist what is best for him.

With our retirees, Jeffrey finally got fed up with going to the bathroom so often and researched on line himself the different options. He decided on the Holmium Light Procedure. Actually the full name is the Holmium Laser Enucleation of the Prostate or HoLEP. This procedure uses a laser to remove tissue blocking urine flow. A separate instrument is then used to cut the prostate tissue into easily removable fragments.

This is similar to prostate surgery that has been used for many years, but requires no incisions. Thus it provides a lasting solution for men with severe prostate problems. For some unknown reason doctors don't suggest this procedure. Jeffrey had to bring it up that he was going to go to the Mayo Clinic to get this done.

Then and only then did his doctor say that his group had someone that did this procedure. So he let them do it and it resolved the problem. It turns out that less than 2% of HoLEP men have to be retreated again for this condition

The good news is that there are several procedures. The bad news is that there are several procedures. It is up to the patient to make the final decision. He should work with his doctor to make this determination, but he not the doctor should make the final decision. Jeffrey made the decision in spite of his doctor and is glad that he did.

Only one of the retirees had cancer of the prostate. He took the procedure that uses radioactive crystals. He has been free of cancer for many years now. People still die from prostate cancer, but most now survive this problem. At this time 99% of prostate cancer patients survive 5 years after surgery. And 90% of localized prostate cancer have complete remission.

Hormone problems affect virtually all women. This is the beginning of menopause and lasts for many years sometimes for life. Katie has been struggling with this since she was in her late

40's. She is now 65 and is still on hormones. She takes Progesterone and Estrogen (Estradiol).

The Progesterone protects the lining of the uterus to keep it from getting too dry. The Estrogen replaces the estrogen hormone that the female produces. It helps with nerves, memory, sleep, hot flashes, etc. All the turmoil that women go through in later years.

There are so many medicines both over the counter and prescribed that have helped some women. It is a crap shoot as to which works for each individual woman. The only way to find the right solution is for each woman to work with her gynecologist to find the best solution for her particular needs. And sometimes you may have to switch gynecologists several times to fine the right combination. Katie switched gynecologists five times before she found the remedy that now works for her.

Some of the remedies can lead to cancer. It is again a crap shoot and a decision each woman has to make. Does she want to be miserable and not worry about cancer? Or does she wish to be comfortable and take her chances? Each woman needs to do her homework and talk to her physician. It may take some experimenting with both remedies and doctors.

Financial

The national average for 67 year olds is $68,905 per year. This compares to our sample at $62,500. In the retirement years beyond 70 the national average was $45,989. This compares to our $44.8k.   So our sample is representative of the total population. These national average numbers were taken from the U.S. Census Bureau's "Current Population Survey".

Interestingly, in our group of ten, the people who are in the best financial category in monthly retirement are the same who walked and have the best health . Which came first the income or the health?

Knowing these people as I do I can state categorically it was the walking, health, and exercise that came first. They didn't do well financially and then decide to walk. They were walking and exercising long before they retired. They just kept it up in retirement.

These retirees still obtain the majority of their income (58%) from Social Security. Roger receives 93.5% of his income from

Social Security, while Gloria receives only 7.4%. Gloria's husband worked at the naval air station where he paid into a government pension rather than social security. Thus he does not get social security. The social security of 7.4% is from the work that Gloria did in her early life.

Retiree	Social Sec.	Pension	Savings	Other
Jeff	73%	26%	0%	1%
Gloria	7.4%	58%	35%	0%
Roger	93.50%	0%	6.50%	0%
Mary	41.40%	0%	42.20%	16.40%
Clete	43.60%	0%	43.40%	13%
Angie	63.7%	15.5%	0%	20.7%
Larry	56.2%	18%	25.8%	0%
Steve	86%	14%	0%	0%
Lottie	42.9%	0%	0%	57.1%
Average	58%	13%	18%	11%

Jeffrey receives the largest pension percent from the company he worked for. His company as well as Larry's, Steve's, and Angie's no longer offer a pension program. They all rely on 401(k)'s for retirement programs. Industrial pensions are basically a thing of the past. Gloria's pension is from her husband's government social security program for his many years of working at the naval air station, but it is called a pension.

Interestingly virtually none of the retirees invested in stocks. Larry did some minor investing during his youth, but it didn't do him much good. He did of course invest in stocks in his 401(k) as did everyone else with a 401(k).

None of the 9 retirees did any serious investing. Jeffrey did purchase 4 rental units and did sell them at a profit and did make some money off the rentals. But he and his wife did not feel it was worth the trouble. So by age 45 they had sold their last unit.

The conventional thinking is that stock equity holdings should be reduced as investors reach retirement. By age 40 investors start to reduce their interest in risky assets. The old adage of "buy low and sell high" would certainly hold water in today's market. Market prices are at an all-time high. So for seniors to invest now would be insane.

How to hedge against inflation is the key to investing. However, there are no truly risk free hedges against inflation. Anyone who buys groceries knows Social Security is not keeping up with inflation.

Seniors do have a major investment in their homes. With interest rates so low, now is the time to refinance your home. If you are paying 4.5% or greater then you can certainly reduce your monthly.

If you have capital in savings, it would make sense to invest in your house by increasing the amount you have in your equity. Jeffrey put $42,000 from his 401(k) into his house mortgage five years ago. He had a 6% mortgage rate at that time. His new mortgage is 3.375% fixed.

By putting $42,000 in his house and refinancing he reduced his monthly almost in half to $888.65. He saved $47,142 over 5 years. So he paid back his initial $42,000 investment and now saves $785.70 per month. The real beauty of this is that the $785.70 is tax free.

He would have to earn approximately $1,047.60 per month to make $785.70 per month. By investing in his house mortgage Jeffrey received 25% (($1,047.60 - $785.70)/1,047.6) per month on just this part of his investment. Beats the heck out of investing in stocks and it is risk free. Plus he saves $9,428.40 (12x$785.70) each year. This is even more significant!

And by having a low mortgage rate more money comes into his equity because he is paying a greater principle ratio. In 5 years Jeffrey has increased his equity by almost exactly $20,000. Plus his house has increased in value over the past 5 years. This was smart investing for a senior on a fixed income. The point is to look at your current market conditions and make a plan.

Plan for the Future

Each senior has to look at his or her position and then make a smart decision. Many seniors downsize their home. They then can have a smaller mortgage and increased cash or both. But be sure that you shop carefully to get the lowest percent and the smallest closing costs. There are pitfalls that need to be accommodated in moving. The section below on moving will cover these.

If a senior is not financially qualified to make a realistic and logical plan then he should work with a reliable and honest financial planner. A planner who does not sell stocks or bonds or has no ulterior motive should be used. Edward Jones calls its people financial planners. Yet their main function is to sell stocks. If they don't sell stocks they won't stay in business.

There is a company called the NAPFA or the National Association of Personal Financial Advisors. Make sure that you obtain someone who specializes in seniors and who handles several people per month. There will be a fee, but it could be worth it. Finding the right planner is imperative.

Your adviser should adhere to the three C's, conflict, competence, and custody. Conflict is misleading. No one is conflict free. You must decide whether to work with a fee-only, a fee based, or commission based.

You should make sure your adviser is competent. You should make sure that your adviser is registered as a financial planner by CFP or the Certified Financial Planner Board of Standards.

You should never never give custody of your assets to your financial adviser. There have been many cases of Ponzi schemes such as the most famous Bernie Madoff situation in which he had control of people's assets.

If you look at the 10 retirees, the five with good plans are the ones who specifically thought out their plans and implemented them. Angie implemented a plan based upon the best she could do at the time. Inflation and repairs will make it difficult for her going forward, but for now she is okay. She had the terrible misfortune of losing her husband when she was young. Jeffrey has a good plan, but he may have to lower his home price to sell it. Larry's plan will carry him for the rest of his life.

Doctors

Doctors can shorten your life, make you comfortable, cost you money, or lengthen your life. It is up to the retiree to control and guide the use of his doctor. Not all doctors are good and not all doctors are bad. Doctors make mistakes. It is up to the retiree to minimize the chance a doctor will screw up the retiree's life.

A retiree should have a good general practitioner. Hopefully, one he has had for many years. One who can direct him to the correct specialist when necessary. But it is still up to the retiree to check out the specialist when the time comes. If a retiree has to have an operation, he better make darn sure that the specialist has performed and performs the procedure routinely and successfully.

A recent example came from my sister in law just this week. She had her deviated septum corrected through surgery. The surgeon told her that she had two problems that he would correct. He would correct the deviated septum and correct the collapsed side of her nose. Apparently as we get older some people's nostrils collapse inward thus cutting proper air flow.

Well the doctor corrected the deviated septum, but neglected to correct the collapsed nostril. He just forgot. So now my sister in law is still in agony and he is going to have to do something to correct this. This is just one example of incompetence in the medical profession. She never checked this doctor's credentials.

It is knowing when to have a procedure and when to just live with it. I have had a deviated septum since I was a teenager playing football. Over the years several doctors have recommended getting it fixed. I have absolutely no plans to ever have it fixed!

Medical

I have separated doctors and medical into two separate entities. Medical is more comprehensive because it includes hospitals and medicines. The most important thing to say about hospitals is to use the biggest and best.

There are plenty of publications that rate hospitals. Several hospitals have clean and sanitized facilities. Not all hospitals do. It is up to the retiree to do this research to select a hospital. How many and what kind of doctors do they have on staff, etc.? How many patients do their nurses handle on shift?   These are just a few of the important questions to ask.

I can relate an experience that happened to me in a hospital that had good doctors on staff. I was having a hernia operation and the doctor and nurse had trouble getting a catheter to go up into my bladder. They kept trying to the point where blood started coming out.

They stopped trying and immediately called a board certified urologist who was on staff. He found out that I had a "flap" or piece of skin that was blocking the catheter. The urologist was able to get around the flap and the operation went on successfully.

It is my personal opinion that there is too much medicine dispersed in this country. Every one of the ten retirees takes at least one medicine every day. Jeffrey takes the least amount and potency. He takes 50 micrograms of Synthroid each day. Most everyone is on either blood thinner or cholesterol medicine or both.

Seventy six percent of all people over 60 take at least two medicines or more each day. Thirty seven percent take five or more. If you are taking five or more this could be the reason that you are feeling just plain lousy.

Prescription medications are increasing among baby boomers and older retirees. Overmedication just creeps up and up. Blood thinners, arthritis medicine, pain medication for backs, sleeping pills, antidepressants, cholesterol medicine, blood pressure medicine, thyroid medicine, opioids for pain and on and on. It's no wonder people don't feel good. Almost half the ads on TV are for one drug or another. They show people enjoying life apparently because they are taking some medicine. But, just listen to the side effects!

So what's the answer? How many of these drugs do you really need? People are scared to stop taking them once they are on them. Doctors scare people. Jeffrey wanted to get off of his Synthroid, but his doctor told him that this could make his skin start to scale.

However, Jeffrey doesn't believe him and has started to reduce his Synthroid. And he feel just fine and hasn't developed scales. He plans to get tested after 6 months of a reduced Synthroid dosage. He will keep reducing it until his test gets out of normal range. What scared Jeffrey was his doctor telling him that once the scaling starts even going back to Synthroid won't stop it. He is still going to continue to reduce taking Synthroid.

The retirees who are doing the walking regiment are the ones who take the least amount of medicine. Maybe walking reduces the need for medicine?   This book is not telling anyone to reduce their medicine, but it is cautioning retirees to work with their doctors to prevent taking too much.

Try to find a doctor who uses common sense over his prescription pad. And ask your doctor if you can safely reduce your amount of medicine. Look up the side effects. Talk to your pharmacist. Go to your doctor specifically for a medication checkup.

Just don't act like sheep when it comes to taking medicine. And for goodness sake start walking. It could just be a block at first. It may feel rough, but keep going. And for sure talk to your doctor before you start a walking program. Try to find a hobby that gets you up and out of your chair. Your chair may be the cause of much of your ailment.

One of the most vicious cycles that happens to retirees is what I call the loss of energy and strength spiral (LESS). The spiral starts with two issues. First, sitting way more than is designed for our bodies. The second is eating more than our bodies are designed for. The more you sit, the more you eat. The more you sit the less strength and energy you have. The more you eat the less energy you have, which causes you to sit more. Thus the spiral.

I shouldn't blame retirees for this problem. Because this problem begins long before people retire. It begins in the mid 30's and 40's. People go to restaurants. The portion size in a restaurant is for 6'6" people with large frames. No one should ever eat the portions put forth by restaurants.

Most people eat the full portions because it is "sinful" to leave food on your plate. Well, just put the "extra" in a "to go" box. All restaurants have these. I do see seniors putting food in boxes, but they are few and far between. My wife and I always put food in "to go" boxes. And many times we split a single meal and still have to put the remains in a "to go" box.

When I go to Cracker Barrel for a meal, I often sit outside in one of their rockers. I enjoy watching the people walk into and out of the restaurant. What catches my attention most is the number of truly obese people. A trim person is a rarity. And Cracker Barrel is a relatively healthy food restaurant.

I would bet that these obese people are the ones who take so much medicine. I would also bet that many of these people are the ones who sit in front of their TV's at night and eat snacks. And these same people are the ones who take the most medicine. This is killing our country and raising the cost of health insurance and health care. Congress can't cure this problem. Okay enough preaching.

Family

Family dynamics is an interesting phenomenon. Who speaks to who and who doesn't speak to whom is the dynamic. However, most families have someone that they truly love and care about. This loving and caring about is what keeps many seniors going.

Grand parenting is a major part of many retirees life. It is interesting to note that in one of my earlier books "Longevity, Living to 120 and Beyond and Enjoying the Ride" nurturing was one of the commonalities of the truly elderly. This nurturing can be to grandchildren and it can be to perfect strangers.

Nurturing does not have to be giving money to grown children or grandchildren. It can be keeping grandchildren while their parents work. This seems to be the most common nurturing performed by grandparents. Chasing a two or three year old will definitely keep you off your sofa or chair.

Those that still have their spouse and enjoy the company of their spouse are the luckiest. But many of the truly elderly have lived for many years alone. It is tougher financially and emotionally.

Downsizing

This is an interesting phenomenon. Most retirees who make a change downsize. But some like Larry actually increased the size of their home after retirement. And some like Larry again actually then went the other direction. In the case of Larry he went from a small house that he lived in most of his life to a much larger house. He then went to a condo that was half the size of his larger house.

But by and large most downsize. They do this for financial reasons mostly. But a two story house can become burdensome in old age. Sure there are motorized stair chairs, but the burden of too much house can be overwhelming. Most women feel the need to clean their house thoroughly. Having an upstairs with children's rooms that are no longer used is unnecessary in most cases.

Excess Stuff

Is your "stuff" controlling you? Think about it. Do you have so many old possessions that you are not using, that you can't think about moving or downsizing. Is your garage so filled with junk that you have to park on the driveway or street? Are you afraid to get rid of "stuff" because you paid good money for it? If yes then you are being controlled by your no longer needed possessions.

The answer is to get rid of "stuff". You will feel better. You will be able to breath. You will be able to move or downsize. So what if you think you are throwing money away. If it is just taking up space then it is robbing you of the space and peace of life. Besides, getting rid of "stuff" can go to those who will truly have a use for it. This is part of nurturing.

It sounds harsh to get rid of stuff and may seem overwhelming. But you can have several garage sales. You can call the salvation army, Goodwill, or any free service that will pick stuff up.

The best part is that you can take something that has been gathering dust in your house, yard, attic, or garage and do good with it. It just may bring joy and happiness and fill a genuine need for someone else. Knowing that you are doing good will make it easier to part with your stuff. And you might just make a little spending money in your garage sale.

And it will cost less when you move.

Best Locations for Retirees

There is no one answer that best describes the best location for retirees. It depends on the needs and wants of the retiree. There are numerous on line reports claiming the best locations for retirees. Unfortunately none of them even have a couple of the same locations in their lists.

Some pick very hot climates like Florida, Arizona, and Texas. While others pick very cold climates like Iowa, Illinois, and Maine. No one can tell a retiree where he should or should not live. Some internet sites recommend foreign countries. Foreign living sounds like something for very young retirees.

For me personally, I have chosen to live in the south. I plan to move to Pensacola, Florida just like Jeffrey. If I could afford it I would live in Pensacola in the fall, winter, and spring and spend summers in the cooler north. Some like Clete did the opposite. He lived spring, summer, and fall in New York State and spent the winter in Florida.

Moving

Whether you are downsizing, building your dream house, or finding a milder climate, the same issues apply when it comes to the actual physical move. Attached Exhibit I covers the basic requirements for the physical move.

The biggest problem comes when you are selling one house and buying another. Coordinating closing times and physical move times is always tricky. It is best if everyone works together and organizes the moving and closing times to everyone's satisfaction.

Reverse Mortgage

Only one of the ten retirees (Angie) in this book obtained a reverse mortgage. For her it was her only logical move. It is certainly not for everyone. But it can be a solution for some.

The way Angie's and most reverse mortgages work is as follows:

1. First you have to select a reputable mortgage company. The biggest is AIG. Angie used Sunset West Mortgage in Cerritos, California. You should shop the best program and rate. Angie used her local credit union to help with the paper work and in deciding on the right company and program.
2. The mortgage company will inspect and assign a value to your home.
3. The value, age of the youngest relative (62 or older) living with you, and equity left in your home will determine the financial arrangement.
4. Basically the mortgage company will pay off your mortgage such that you no longer make mortgage payments. Angie used to pay $707.72 and now has no payment to make.
5. You or any relative living with you are entitled to remain in your home until the last relative living with you is deceased. There is an age factor here. The youngest

member in your house has to be of sufficient age like 62 to qualify for the reverse mortgage.

6. You next have a choice to make. The reverse mortgage company will give you a choice. You can have equity to draw from that increases at a specified rate of interest. Or you can have a monthly check. In Angie's case she chose the equity, which amounts to $29,366 this month. It grew from the previous month by $108.00 or roughly 3.7%. If she had chosen the monthly income she would have gotten $145 per month. Basically, the choices for anyone are:

    a. As a lump sum in cash, at settlement
    b. As an annuity, with a monthly cash payment
    c. As a line of credit, similar to a home equity line of credit. Angie chose this.

7. As a combination lump sum and annuity, with a smaller lump sum at settlement and then a smaller annuity.
8. In Angie's case when she dies her heirs have one year to empty the house. They could also buy the house from the mortgage company. If they did nothing but remove the contents then the mortgage company takes over the house.
9. If there is anything left in the equity account it goes to Angie's heirs.
10. Where the property sells for more than the amount owed to the lender, the borrower or their estate will receive the extra funds. However, the borrower (retiree's estate) cannot be charged if the house sells for less than is owed.

In calling several mortgage companies, it looks like the equity loan is approximately 20% of the equity in the house. This number varies by the lowest age of the retirees in the house. But it does not vary significantly.

The negative to the reverse mortgage is the fact that the retiree is somewhat stuck in his or her house. He can't sell it without paying off what he "owes" to the reverse mortgage company.

Anyway it is a serious option for any retiree with a limited income. Recent legislation has made it even better as follows:

1. Under the National Credit Code penalties for early repayment are illegal on new loans since September 2012, however a bank may charge a reasonable administration fee for preparation of the discharge of mortgage.
2. Also in 2012, the government introduced statutory 'negative equity protection' on all new reverse mortgage contracts. You cannot end up owing the lender more than your home is worth (the market value or equity).

Investing

There are so many companies wanting your money to invest that it is scary. Just remember no one is in it for your benefit as much as their benefit. The worst thing a retiree can do is try to make a fortune by depriving themselves of enjoying their remaining years. For instance, if you have $300,000 in savings and you are 75 then-- It would make more sense to spend this money than trying to save it to make more.

There are retirees that deprive themselves of a yearly vacation because they don't want to pull money out of their stocks. If you have $300,000 and you are 75, you should plan on spending at least $10,000 per year on vacation. Saving this money or worse putting it into a risky stock portfolio would make no sense. In other words, invest in yourself.

There are so many low risk investments that it would take too much space to go into. But be sure whatever you invest in provides the option to get your money within 24 hours of requesting. Also, be darned sure that no one has control of your investment but you. Remember Bernie Maddox!

How do You Compare to Other Retirees?

You have been able to compare yourself to the 9 retirees in this book. Nationally other retirees have the following statistics:

1. Average age of retiring from working --------------- 63
2. Average length of retirement ----------------------- 18
3. Cost of couple's medical treatment past 65 -----$218,000
4. Percentage over 65 relying completely on S.S.   36%
5. Percentage who don't save anything for retiring 38%

6. Percentage of population over 65 ----------------- 13%
7. By age 65 the number considered wealthy ------- 1%
8. By age 65 the number who have adequate capital 4%
9. By age 65 retirees who will still be working ----- 3%
10. By 65 those depending on S.S., friends, relatives, 63%
11. Those that have died by 65 ------------------------ 29%
12. Amount Medicare covers of average medical ---- 62%
13. One year of skilled nursing care in a facility -- $200,000
14. Average household income of 67 year olds--- $68,905
15. Beyond 70 the average household income ----$45,989
16. Median (1/2 above) income household @ 75 - $30,635

Beginning in the year 2034 Social Security will have run out of money and only be able to afford to cover 77% of promised benefits. I have to believe that our government won't let this happen. However, no one knows for sure what our government will do. However, by 2034 retirees will be a larger percentage of the population. They should be able to control what happens to them.

Retirees need to ban together as a political force. One of the biggest problems besides inflation affecting retirees is property taxes. I believe that when a person reaches 66 his tax bill for property should be frozen at the then price. It should not keep going up each year.

As anyone who purchases groceries knows, inflation is growing far more rapidly than our social security benefits are increasing. Retirees need to become a major political force. Until that happens retirees are going to continue to get put upon.

They will have to cut back on everything from food to clothing to housing. There are currently over 100 retiree website blogs that are put out by many different sources. Just go on line and put "websites for retirees" in the search window. But try to enjoy the rest of your life. Just don't sit in a chair and vegetate. And remember to walk, walk, walk.

My personal best regards to my fellow retirees,

John D. Forlini

Exhibit 1
(Moving Check List)

<u>Moving from Current Address</u>

1. Cancel:
    - Mail-Use new forwarding address
    - Electricity
    - Gas
    - Water & Sewage
    - Garbage
    - Newspaper
    - Termite bond
    - Lawn service

2. Transfer from Current Address to New Address
    - Cable or TV service
    - Internet service
    - Church Affiliation
    - Banks
    - Check address
    - Driver's licenses
    - Car tags
    - Professional licenses
    - Telephone (land line and/or cell)
    - Car insurance
    - House insurance

3. Physical Move
    - Professional or
    - Self-Move
    - Pods

Cancelling is straight forward. Transferring is not necessarily so simple. For instance, if your bank receives income from sources and it does not have a branch office in the new state you are moving to, then you have several options.

For instance, Jeffrey will be moving from Alabama to Florida. He is lucky that his income from Social Security, pension fund, and royalties goes into a bank that has branches in Florida. He just has to have his checks with new addresses.

On the other hand Larry does not have a branch office in North Carolina. He has two choices. He can notify all those putting income into his current bank of a new bank and routing etc. or he can continue with his bank in Alabama. If he does then he has to make arrangements to either bank by internet, mail, or some other means or utilize two different banks and make transfers.

State professional licenses such as real estate and insurance licenses must have notification to the state of origin if these licenses are to remain in effect. Some states have reciprocal license arrangements. In this case the license may be transferred. In Jeffrey's case he will transfer his Alabama real estate license to Florida. He only has 30 days to notify Alabama of this change of address. He must also take several hours of training in Florida to complete the transfer.

There are three main methods of moving. I have personally used professional moving companies two out of my 14 moves. Both of these were paid for by the companies I was working for. I could not have afforded them otherwise.

In my other 12 moves I hired 2-4 people to load the truck with furnishings from my current address and then 2-4 to unload at the new address. Three times the moves were in the same area and I was able to use the same crew for both load and unload.

Doing it myself was actually less hassle. The professionals tended to want to just get it moving and weren't patient with our positioning of items or putting things together properly.

We used medium sized boxes, some small, and very little large boxes. The smaller boxes were easier to handle. All 14 moves were good. My wife is very organized and a good packer. We labelled the boxes on the top and on the side. We took pictures of each of our current rooms before removing furniture. We tried to load one room at a time. The professional movers did not like this idea. Going up in square footage was considerably better for moving. Downsizing always created problems.

Labor for loading and unloading was obtained from several sources. The local Pensacola shopper was a good source for our three moves in Pensacola. The labor for our three moves in the Birmingham area came from our local Mexican population. The Mexicans stood on a certain corner waiting to be hired. They were some of the best of movers, but we did not have bad movers in any of our moves. The state unemployment office is another source of labor.